SMOKER

Self-Portrait of a Nicotine Addict

ELLEN WALKER

1817

A Harper/Hazelden Book

Harper & Row, Publishers, San Francisco

New York, Grand Rapids, Philadelphia, St. Louis
London, Singapore, Sydney, Tokyo, Toronto

For Dad

FIRST HARPER & ROW EDITION PUBLISHED IN 1990.

Library of Congress Cataloging-in-Publication Data

Walker, Ellen.
    Smoker : self-portrait of a nicotine addict / Ellen Walker.—1st Harper & Row ed.
        p.   cm.
    "A Harper/Hazelden book."
    Reprint. Originally published: Center City, MN : Hazelden, 1989.
    Includes bibliographical references.
    ISBN 0-06-255390-9
    1. Walker, Ellen.   2. Cigarette smokers—United States—Biography.
3. Cigarette habit—United States.   I. Title.
HF5731.5.W35A3   1990
362.29′6′092—dc20   89-83561
                                                    CIP

ISBN 0-06-255390-9 (pbk.)

90 91 92 93 94 MUR 10 9 8 7 6 5 4 3 2 1

Contents

Foreword

This book is unique in that it is the first time Hazelden has published anything about being addicted to a specific drug or behavior, in this case nicotine, where the author is a practicing addict. All our other materials are written by people who, at least at the time of publication, are understood to be in recovery from addiction to the drug or behavior they are writing about. The only exception to this are the works by treatment professionals or professional writers who, while not necessarily in a recovery program themselves, are assumed not to be practicing addicts.

The reason for this unwritten policy is simple. Our mission is and always has been to support, reinforce, and nurture our readers' Twelve Step recovery programs. To us this has meant conveying the experience, strength, and hope of those who have recovered their sanity and honesty through total abstinence.

And yet, assuming that our authors are a fairly representative sampling of people in recovery programs, it is safe to say that a good percentage of them were using the drug nicotine while they were writing these materials for us. A visit to most Twelve Step meetings and drug treatment centers will confirm the prevalence of nicotine use by people, including treatment counselors, who otherwise are abstinent from mood-altering chemicals and consider themselves recovering.

This is not to point a finger but simply to illustrate how uniquely this drug is still regarded in the recovery community, not to mention our culture at large. While few would dispute that nicotine is a powerfully addictive chemical, few also apply the same standards to it as to drugs with a fraction of nicotine's destructiveness and prevalence.

This is exactly the contradiction that Ellen Walker describes so eloquently in this book and, in fact, embodies in her personal struggle as a smoker. Filled with insight into the addictive process, cognizant of her powerlessness over nicotine, still she smokes. It is almost as if she and the many other tobacco users like her (and their enablers?) are dangling in the middle of the First Step. They are well aware of their powerlessness over their "drug of choice" but are still in the process of defining what unmanageability is, short of the many debilitating and fatal illnesses that tobacco can eventually cause.

It seemed to me, considering the unprecedented crisis point so many of us are at with this uniquely cunning, baffling, powerful drug, that this was a story worth making an exception for. This isn't meant as a self-help book but more a dramatic portrayal of how things are now for one woman who may be representative of the many millions trapped by this insidious chemical.

Of course, thousands of other nicotine addicts have already begun their journey of recovery with total abstinence, one day at a time. We have and will continue to tell their stories, too, as evidenced by *If Only I Could Quit* by Karen Casey. In the back of this book is an appendix reprinted from our pamphlet, *Twelve Steps for Tobacco Users*, by Jeanne E., a short guide to utilizing cessation and recovery methods and programs. These programs have helped many recovering tobacco users and will help even more in the future as understanding and acceptance of this illness grow.

I join with Ellen in the hope that this book contributes to that process.

THE EDITOR

Acknowledgments

Even a book such as this, so filled with personal experiences and private feelings, is the product of more than one person. Dozens of other smokers—close friends and perfect strangers—have encouraged me to honestly discuss our addiction to nicotine. My family members, too, have supported me in my decision to identify myself as an addict and my smoking behavior as an illness. Hazelden editor, Sid Farrar, has been unwavering in his belief in the topic. He has generously given his time and expertise to this project. Thank you all.

For thy sake, tobacco, I
would do anything but die.
— Charles Lamb

THE LUCK OF THE DRAW

The End of a Life

His alcoholism was killing him, just as we had always feared it would. Cirrhosis of the liver, the doctor had told us. But there was a glimmer of hope. If our father would stop drinking, his liver could repair itself. His doctor assured us we would see almost immediate improvement. With that brightening news, Dad went home resolving to never take another drink.

Home again, he rested, ate nourishing meals, and was abstinent; but his condition worsened. He was increasingly tired and, despite family members' pleas to eat more, he ate less and less. Instead, he slept. The doctor responded to our worried phone calls with assurance. Perhaps we were being too impatient, he said, but soon we should see improvement if Dad was, in fact, abstinent.

Within two weeks, my father had become so weak he had to be physically supported by my stepmother as he made more and more frequent trips to the bathroom. My husband and I visited with them a couple days after Christmas, and my stepmother pulled me aside to voice her concerns. "He's not getting better," she said. "I think he's a lot worse. Don't you?" We called his doctor, and again we were assured that Dad's tiredness was probably his body's attempt to rest and heal itself.

Two days later, when we went to their home again, he was clearly a seriously ill man. He slept almost constantly. And when we did rouse him, his pasty coloration and wide-eyed, almost puzzled, gaze were that of a stranger. My husband said quietly, "Call an ambulance," and when we explained to Dad he was going back to the hospital, he nodded and offered no argument.

The lab tests done during his last hospital stay finally produced some answers. My brother and I sat down with one

3

of his doctors after Dad had been in the hospital for six days. The tests, he explained to us, only now were producing a diagnosis. "Your father is dying of cancer," he told us. The cancer growth was literally supplanting his liver. The cancer had originated elsewhere; it was an oat-cell cancer of the lung which had metastasized and established itself in the liver. The doctor was tender, gentle, but he was also clear in his statement that our father could live no more than a few days.

We walked back to Dad's room and stood on each side of his bed. I touched his arm repeatedly to rouse him as we tried to talk to him. Our words seemed so inappropriate—my brother's job, our children's comings and goings, even the weather—meaningless would be a better word. We never were sure if he heard or understood because we could awaken him for only a few seconds before his eyes closed again. Occasionally he would sigh as though in reply.

In his last days, Dad's weariness made him incapable of little, other than sleep and an occasional mumbled question, much like the sounds of a small child unexpectedly drifting off to sleep. He could accept only a few spoonfuls of food. Unable to accept the reality of his condition, we continued to push food at him, clinging to the belief that nourishment could heal him.

Mostly, we watched. Slowly we began to accept that he would die here, that there was nothing we could do, and that we could even be thankful that his death would not be the agony of many cancer victims. We would awaken him from time to time to once more make contact, but mostly we watched. And what we saw was a man whose functioning had eroded to instinct only.

Throughout his hospital stay, he repeated an instinctive motion several times each hour. Even when he became too exhausted to eat, talk, or respond to our conversations, he continued to make this gesture. His right hand would rise to his face, and at first it seemed as though he were trying to merely touch his nose with his middle finger. This nonsensical motion finally made sense to me: "He thinks he's smoking," I told the others.

Oat-cell cancer of the lung, the cancer that led to my father's death, is virtually unknown among nonsmokers. It was smoking that killed him—fifty-five years of two or more packs a day. The ultimate irony is that the only instinct, perhaps the only comfort, left him as he lay dying of cancer was smoking. This once powerful man, now stripped of vitality and personality, this man who couldn't pull himself out of his lethargy to respond to loved ones, was so physically and mentally driven by nicotine that any energy he had was used to recreate a robot-like smoking behavior. It was obscene.

It was obscene but easily explained. The fact is, there was probably no other action or behavior my father performed as frequently as smoking. It was a constant presence in his life. Although none of us realized it then, he had no more control over where or when he smoked than he did over the nicotine-seeking movements he made lying in his hospital bed. He was addicted to nicotine, and like all addicts he had lost control over the substance. Years earlier, the addiction had become the driver of his life. It continued to be till the moment of his death.

* * *

Not Just Statistics

It's hard for those untouched by a disease like nicotine addiction to see the human element of it. They see the numbers. What is the total cost of medical treatment for tobacco users? What is their absentee rate at work? How does it affect the cost of consumer goods or insurance rates? Or they see the results of the addicts' compulsive use—a pile of cigarette butts carelessly strewn on a parking lot, a devastating forest fire, the stains in public buildings.

But the souls of addicts don't show. It's nearly impossible for a nonaddict to know the self-deprecation, frustration, and fear of those who are held in the grip of nicotine. Yet, we are talking about people.

I thought I understood my father's alcoholism. I'd seen him once before in a hospital after hip surgery, and in his eyes I'd seen a frightened little boy. He looked so vulnerable and unprotected. That view of him gave me an idea of why he sought comfort in alcohol. Some time later, I confronted him about his drinking and asked him to quit. "It could kill you," I told him.

"I don't know," he said. "Nah. But do you know what will kill me? These." And he gestured with the ever-present cigarette.

On the day of his funeral, I remembered his prediction. And I wondered then, as I do even now, how much of the vulnerability and fear I'd once seen was due to withdrawal from nicotine, rather than from alcohol. After all, it's rare for an alcoholic to maintain a constant state of inebriation, but most tobacco users seek a steady level of nicotine in their system. My father didn't drink every day, but—except for a few attempts to quit—he smoked every day for fifty-five years. He smoked hundreds of thousands of cigarettes; more than six million times he surrendered to the nearly instantaneous relief—the hit—of inhaling that warm chemical mixture.

To most people my father was just a statistic in 1982, along with the hundreds of thousands of others who died of tobacco-related causes that year. But these were *people*—husbands, wives, fathers, mothers, and even children—people whose lives were shortened needlessly ("I wish I could have two more years with you," my father had told his wife), people whose deaths were mourned by those left behind.

My two brothers, my sister, and I were scattered among the many people who had gathered in the church basement after the funeral. Increasingly, I felt agitated as I nodded in acceptance of expressions of sympathy. Grief had weakened me; I felt out of control. We had been there for almost two hours. Across the room, the minister was talking with one of the active church members, and suddenly I was aware of the anger I felt toward him. He had dispatched my father in record time, using the stock Scripture passages and not once saying Dad's name. There was shame, too, that Dad was a stranger here, that we all were.

A longtime friend of my dad, a drinking companion, shyly approached me and said he was sorry. Then he asked the question whose answer he feared: "What did the autopsy say?" A bizarre answer leaped into my mind. I wanted to tell the man, "It said he was dead," but I held back these bitter words.

"He had cancer," I told him, and relief spread across his face. I could well imagine the fear he had that cirrhosis had killed my father. Cancer, however, kept this man safe from facing the dangers of his own alcoholism.

I had to get out of there before I said or did something I'd regret. A wave of reality hit me: my dad was dead, and his death was not only a loss but a threat. No longer was there a full generation of people between me and my death.

A silent understanding passed among my siblings and me. We walked up the stairs together and out the back door into a bitter, cold January day. The northwest wind whipped at us as we hugged each other and cried. I mechanically cupped my hands and turned my back against the wind to protect the flame of my lighter as I lit my cigarette. Ritualistically, we all leaned our heads back to exhale with breathy sighs. In a matter of seconds, my erratic thoughts and out-of-control emotions settled back neatly into ordered calmness. We said little as we stood there, four dark figures against the January snow. But I knew nothing really had to be said. Everything was all right.

* * *

"Kind of "a Drug

Cigarettes and other tobacco products have been accepted as part of our culture for so long it's difficult for us to think of them as addictive. Until fairly recently, they were widely held to have many positive attributes. Early users not only were ignorant of the health risks but actually believed tobacco had certain medicinal benefits. Even today, with the widespread evidence of diseases related to tobacco use, it's common to hear people say that smoking relaxes them or increases their concentration.

Tobacco use—especially by pipe and cigarette smokers—is often accepted as part of their personas by virtue of how and what they smoke. A close look at movies bears this out. A pipe smoker often is depicted as studious or highly intelligent. The Bogart squint with cigarette in mouth is understood as a sign of strength and independence. The manner in which the performer smokes helps moviegoers identify the bad guy, the hero, the temptress, even the fool. Smoking is a theatrical device which moves the plot forward: the lighting of a cigarette could be a sexual overture or a further definition of the character's strength or insecurity; the manner in which the actor extinguishes a cigarette can convey anything from anger, to decisiveness, to fear.

Tobacco advertisers also employ these devices to sell their products. Publication and billboard advertisements are saturated with the message that this or that cigarette is used by active people. By sexually attractive people. By strong, independent people. Despite the health warnings on the ads, the messages ring out clearly, and they're seen by the people who are most vulnerable—preteens and teenagers. Older people are not likely to be swayed by these ads. If they don't smoke, they're not apt to begin. If they do, they've already made a commitment to a brand and will probably change only if they believe one is "healthier" than another. But the young are susceptible to these messages because many of them are plagued with a self-doubt that makes them easy prey to the empty promises of personal strength, attractiveness, and self-sufficiency coming from companies producing cigarettes or perfume or designer jeans. But there is a difference between these products: At the age of twenty-five or thirty, people can choose to discard jeans or discontinue use of perfume, but those who use tobacco often can't make that choice. For many, by that time, the dynamics of nicotine addiction have removed that option. They might throw out the blue jeans, but they'll check the pockets for cigarettes first.

Addiction may seem to be a drastic or extreme word to describe tobacco use. After all, many people have tried tobacco once and never used it again. To them, the continued use by others may seem to be a repeated choice to experience the horrible taste and sick feelings that they remember from their brief exposure to tobacco. Or the word *addiction* may evoke only images of needle-using addicts, death from overdose, violence, and a high crime rate to meet the exorbitant cost of keeping supplied. Yet, comparative studies of heroin and nicotine show similarities in the addictive process at work — from the drive to use to the severity of withdrawal. Certainly, there are differences. The cost of most illicit drugs contributes to violent crimes, whereas we don't hear of smokers knocking off a bank to support their drug habit. The most costly difference to smokers, though, is an annual death toll of nearly 390,000. A shocking figure when compared to the 4,000 heroin-related deaths each year.

We resist labeling nicotine as addictive. After all, we've lived our lives with nicotine being used openly and unashamedly. Perhaps we've been so bombarded with ads and movies that we can't see tobacco use as an abnormal means to ingest a drug. It's been such a normal part of American life, how can it be abnormal?

Even those of us who fully believe nicotine to be a dangerous addictive substance sometimes revert to our old notions. It's so easy to say, "Yes, it's definitely addictive," and with the next breath imply that tobacco users should be able to quit more easily than other addicts. Years of conditioning seem to tell us that heroin and alcohol are serious drugs but nicotine is "kind of" a drug. With that mind-set, we have become part of the problem by not offering the support and expertise to smokers in their attempts to quit and by implying to young people that the lure of tobacco doesn't have serious consequences.

Some compulsive traits are shared by all addicts, including nicotine users. Dr. Stephen J. Levy, in his book, *Managing the Drugs in Your Life,* discusses some of those similarities:

> Cigarette smokers have something in common with heroin addicts, speed freaks, garbage heads, and alcoholics: their addiction is a way of life. Smokers overdose . . . they go through some heavy-duty withdrawal . . . and generally tend to adopt behaviors that go along with any addiction: protecting their supply, borrowing money or cigarettes, sneaking cigarettes, lying to themselves and others about stopping, feeling they can't enjoy life without their drug, and using all the other rationalizations and defenses needed to explain away a dangerous and life-threatening habit. Smokers learn to ignore the pleas of loved ones, they learn to deny their own objective medical symptoms, they learn to lie and manipulate . . . and so on.

In the past fifteen years, considerable research has been done to identify and understand the dynamics of nicotine addiction. The 1988 surgeon general's report on smoking devoted itself entirely to nicotine addiction and summaries of nicotine addiction research. At the core of the report's findings are the following statements:

1. Cigarettes and other forms of tobacco are addicting.
2. Nicotine is the drug in tobacco that causes addiction.
3. The pharmacologic and behavioral processes that determine tobacco addiction are similar to those that determine addiction to drugs such as heroin and cocaine.

Reports from the surgeon general in earlier years had stated that nicotine was addictive, but these findings were not the major focus of those reports. They were, instead, secondary to the primary topics, such as cancer (1982 report), cardiovascular disease (1983), and lung disease (1984). The 1988 surgeon general's report, however, was totally dedicated to the exploration of tobacco use and the addictive properties of nicotine. One major conclusion, with the substantiation of 171 research studies conducted by more than 50 eminent scientists, was this: TOBACCO PRODUCTS, NO MATTER HOW THEY ARE INTRODUCED INTO THE BODY, ARE ADDICTING BECAUSE OF THE NICOTINE THEY ALL CONTAIN.

The release of the report was given substantial play in the media. For a brief time, no day passed without exposing the public to newspaper, TV, and radio interviews with the experts. They were everywhere, as were articles, programs, and graphics chronicling the history of nicotine use or touting how-to-quit strategies.

And then nothing. Nicotine as an addiction was no longer news. But nicotine as an addiction *is* news because very few people have accepted it as fact, many smokers included. They continue to view tobacco use, especially smoking, simply as an irritating, selfish habit. They believe nicotine use to be a matter of choice, and quitting to be a simple act of choosing not to smoke.

The prevailing attitude has been one of "anyone can quit

who really wants to." Despite research conclusions, some as early as the 1920s and 1930s, that tobacco products are addictive, many of us have refused to change our opinions of nicotine products. By not accepting the fact of nicotine addiction, we are locked into other unchanging attitudes:

- We can convince users, young and old alike, to quit to protect their health.
- Tobacco users deserve the consequences to their health because they've deliberately ignored the "facts."
- We can legislate ourselves into a smoke-free society by not allowing users to smoke in public areas and workplaces.
- If I can quit, anyone can quit.
- Tobacco users are insensitive, selfish people who ignore the welfare and wishes of others by choosing to use (especially, to smoke) in disallowed areas and at inappropriate times.

It's universally known that continued use of tobacco products substantially increases the odds that the user will die prematurely. Lung cancer and mouth cancer are often cited as the threats to the user's life, but emphysema, heart disease, stroke, pancreatic cancer, and a myriad of other diseases also strike down nicotine addicts with more frequency than nonusers. It has been known for some time that newborns and nursing infants of smoking mothers have measurable levels of nicotine in their systems, that infant birth weight is significantly lowered by nicotine, and that it raises the rate of stillborn and infant mortality. Yet people like me continue to use cigarettes, pipes, or smokeless tobacco. What are these people thinking about? How can they ignore the fact that their choice to continue using tobacco decreases their life expectancy as well as the quality of that life?

I'll answer for myself. I don't choose to continue; I am compelled to continue by an addiction, by a drug that has taken control of my life. As with other addictions, a drug often dictates where I go, which people I associate with, even where

I will work. Nicotine addiction has also locked me into the same patterns of denial which has imprisoned people addicted to other drugs.

There are fifty-five million of us smokers in America alone. Each year, about 40 percent of us attempt to quit. Most of us are unsuccessful. This is not "kind of" a problem, no more than nicotine is "kind of" addictive. This drug is a powerful, at times overwhelming, force in the lives of many of us tobacco users. As with any other drug, addiction to nicotine is a disease of the body, mind, and spirit. It creates a physical and psychological dependence equal to or greater than any other drug; it lets the spirit wither.

* * *

Why Do They Start?

She knew nothing of addiction when she graduated that May; even her father's heavy drinking had no formal name. An alcoholic was a perpetual drunk, a stranger, someone far away, not someone nearby who in an instant could leap from a quiet gentleness to terrifying rage.

If she thought of her father at all as she impatiently waited for those summer days to pass, it was with increasing coolness. His streaks of meanness didn't affect her the way they once had. She was no longer fooled by his deliberate attempts to feign kindness and love, only to crush his unsuspecting victims. She knew the plan, the pattern, and knowing it was a protection. Although she was barely seventeen, she knew how to take care of herself.

High school had been the happiest part of life to date, and she was confident the college years ahead would be a mere extension of those in high school—activities, friends, and success. She used the summer to say good-bye to the farm and to her friends, to prepare for college, and to accustom herself to the freedom of adulthood. There were no doubts she'd do well. After all, hadn't her teachers assured her of that? ("With your IQ, you can be or do anything you want," one had said. "With your personality, you'll have no problem making friends in college," said another.)

So, armed with intelligence, personality, and a wardrobe of old clothes augmented by a new skirt and sweater set, two blouses, and two gathered skirts she'd made, she set off to become a math teacher. She was not armed well enough.

The expectation of continued success had been based on the past: the gentle pace of farm living, effortless achievement in a class of twenty-seven, the safety of a small community. College, she discovered, was not like that. Since she had tested out of the basic required math classes, she registered for an advanced course. For her, the class was like being unexpectedly thrown into a second-year Spanish class. The book had foreign-looking phrases and symbols. Sets? She knew nothing of them, and for the first time in her life she struggled, failed, and struggled some more in the classroom. By the end of her first year, she tossed the dream of a math major aside as unimportant and chose instead a major in English.

The assortment of clothes, so impressive looking when laid out in the living room at home, was sparse and inadequate here. Most girls, at least those she thought of as popular, had many—sometimes dozens—of coordinated outfits. They owned several pairs of shoes and often wore nylons rather than bobby socks. One group, who belonged to a sorority for which she'd never qualify, prided themselves on wearing gloves outdoors at all times. She felt ugly, dumb, and alone. The isolation was even greater on her visits home because she had to protect herself with an armor of pretense that everything was fine.

The college, in the mode of the late fifties and early sixties, believing its responsibility to extend beyond mere education, sponsored "teas" twice a year. The girl's first tea was a disaster. Everyone was to wear hats, she was told. Another girl in her dorm offered one of hers (she had several). And gloves! Another girl let her borrow an extra pair. Adorned with the bounty of others, she fearfully attended the tea ("Your presence is required"). Later, she could never be sure whether her social blunders at the tea were due to true ignorance or just nervousness. Years would go by before she could see any humor in the Fall Tea Caper, as she called it. It would take that much time before she could find more amusement than pain in remembering how she took the cup *and* saucer, rather than just the cup, as protocol dictated. Worse still was her embarrassment over being caught holding her cake in her gloved hand and eating from it much as she would have done back home.

An old, familiar feeling had eased upon her almost from the beginning – a sense of being different. She had almost forgotten that terrifying feeling of being without friends, of being alone. It had been so long ago, and now – like then – she felt helpless. Being vulnerable and frightened was not acceptable, so she adapted and, as easily as she had with her major, she discarded the old self – the brain, the athlete. She worked like a performer to create a new personality acceptable to those new people around her. She was funny, even outrageous, trying desperately to find acceptance and friends. The acceptance of one group was finally offered, and she grasped it.

She discovered this group one day by accident when she took a different route from the mailbox to her room. A familiar aroma filled the air as she walked along the basement hallway, and the sound of friendly, bantering voices drew her into the doorway of "B" smoker. For the rest of the year, this room became a haven for her, a safe place where she could always find acceptance and comradery. She felt like a child among these seemingly older girls; yet they were all the same age. A bonding action occurred as they shared their cigarettes with her. During her first weeks in this new society, the girl was often given sample packs of Winstons by another girl who refused payment for them, saying, "Oh, I get them free. I'm just supposed to share them." Within this room, the girl discovered her identity. She belonged; she had become a smoker.

Nonsmokers often express amazement that anyone ever starts smoking or using other tobacco products. "Why do they start?" they ask. Smokers themselves wonder too. Years later, after having smoked for fifteen or more years, she would wonder if she would have become a smoker if she'd gone to college elsewhere. Or if the college she did choose had had a new dormitory for freshmen. Because the dormitory in which the girl lived was old, the girls were restricted from using most electrical appliances and from smoking in their rooms. The freshmen who smoked had to do so in either the "A" smoker or the "B" smoker, depending whether they lived in the A or B wing of the dorm.

There is no way to know for certain that this caused or allowed the girl to become a smoker. Perhaps it did, but then again maybe she was genetically destined to become an addict. Or maybe she had some sort of chemical imbalance that caused those feelings, an imbalance that was miraculously balanced by nicotine. Or was it a learned behavior? Had she learned in her family of origin to handle stress, fear, and pain with a drug?

Decades later, the woman—hating the addiction, but unable to quit—asked herself the questions smokers have been asking for years: *Why did I start? Why can't I quit?* She thought about the girl she once was and the woman she was now. And then she knew. Being vulnerable was unacceptable. Oh, there may be a hundred other reasons, but this is the one she saw clearly. At seventeen, she had felt lonely—and was comforted by nicotine. She had felt afraid—and nicotine masked her fear. She had felt weak—and nicotine gave her the illusion of strength.

Her friends, the woman thought, would be shocked to hear her describe herself as an addict. They might even point to her successes, to how normal she was, to how unlike an addict she was. But they could only see the outside; she knew the inside. She was touched by compassion for the little girl who strode off so unprepared those many years ago, who found a simple way to handle vulnerability and pain.

Why do they start using nicotine? Simple. Nicotine changes the unbearable to the bearable, anger to calmness, fear to courage. It diminishes sadness and pain. Why don't they stop? It suddenly was so clear. Nicotine does everything asked of it. It works.

* * *

We're So Normal

No one nearby would have any trouble identifying my addiction as a problem if I were crazy acting, abusive, or otherwise out of control. As it is, I appear to be in control when I'm smoking and don't exhibit any wild personality changes. Maybe all of us smokers are too normal. Except for being compelled to light up at regular intervals, we look and act like nonsmokers. If there are no other addictions, no other mental illness, and no major family problems, we can easily pass ourselves off as normal in every way. Our lives seem orderly, productive, and autonomous.

Recently I was talking with two nonsmokers who told about their experimentation with smoking. "I remember really feeling high," said one, and the other nodded. This intrigued me, and I asked them to describe the high. What they mentioned—lightheadedness, dizziness, a swimming sensation—are probably common to all first-time smokers and are just symptoms of mild nicotine poisoning. But they both said they remembered a euphoria, and this puzzled me.

"Didn't you have that feeling?" one asked. I hadn't. I recall some dizziness but certainly never felt high. In fact, listening to them made me realize that cigarettes have never made me feel high; they make me feel *normal*. It's possible I don't remember those first experimental drags, so all I can judge is how I feel now when I smoke. And how I feel now is normal—at least what I *think* is normal.

Normal to me means calm. It means not being afraid. Smoking removes the most angry or saddening thoughts from my mind. When I smoke, I can forget—really forget—my mistakes and weaknesses, hunger, or tiredness. It gives me a peace that I've found no place else. If it were a prescription drug, I'd proclaim it a miracle. None of this did I tell my friends because I know this kind of thinking isn't . . .

normal. Knowing this made me uncomfortable, and I knew exactly what to do about that; I reached for my cigarettes.

It always amazes me when nonsmokers describe their youthful experimentation with cigarettes. "Boy," they'll say, "I tried it a few times with some friends, and I just hated the taste. I felt dizzy and sick. I decided right then and there, it wasn't for me." By implication, what they're saying is, "I'm not like you; I chose not to smoke." But by saying they, too, tried cigarettes, they're saying that I'm really no different from them. Like them, I tried smoking with some friends. I, too, hated the taste, got dizzy, felt sick. And, just like these nonsmokers, I "knew" I'd never become a smoker. I made a conscious decision to smoke only when I was with my new smoking friends and swore that the first time I didn't get dizzy I would stop. It never occurred to me I was taking a risk because I really thought I was in control.

This type of thinking is characteristic of young people. Many of us tried smoking then, just as we screamed around corners and pushed our cars to dangerous speeds. Our parents' warnings of what-ifs ("What if a tire would blow out?" "What if a car were approaching on the other side of the hill?" "What if the brakes went out?") went unheeded. We were young. Nothing could happen to us. We knew how to handle loaded guns. The jack would hold while we crawled under the car. For young people, the list of risks taken is nearly endless: fooling with knives, climbing trees, having sex, experimenting with drugs. Risk taking was no risk to us because it (car accidents, gunshot wounds, pregnancies) would never happen to us.

I feel anger toward these people who told me they chose not to continue smoking. I want to tell them, "Well, do you think I chose to smoke? Do you believe I took a cigarette and said, 'I think I'll smoke this one and then maybe four hundred thousand more'? I'm just like you, except you were lucky. We both chose to smoke a few cigarettes, except you never lost your power to choose. I lost that power. I don't know when—I don't even remember noticing that smoking no longer made me dizzy. It really doesn't matter because by then, my luck had probably run out."

* * *

Passing the Test

Smokers Anonymous publishes a checklist to help smokers and their families determine if they are addicted to nicotine. I've written down my answers to the questions. You may want to see how you fare too.

What Are the Symptoms?

Answer the following questions as honestly as you can:

1. Do you smoke every day?

   Yes

2. Do you smoke because of shyness and to build up self-confidence?

   Yes

3. Do you smoke to escape from boredom and worries or while under pressure?

   Yes

4. Have you ever burned a hole in your clothes, carpet, furniture, or car?

   Yes

5. Have you ever had to go to the store late at night or at another inconvenient time because you were out of cigarettes?

   Yes

6. Do you feel defensive or angry when people tell you that your cigarette smoke is bothering them?

yes

7. Has a doctor or dentist suggested that you stop smoking?

yes

8. Have you promised someone that you would stop smoking, then broken your promise?

yes

9. Have you felt physical or emotional discomfort when trying to quit?

yes

10. Have you successfully stopped smoking for a period of time only to start again?

yes

11. Do you buy extra supplies of tobacco to make sure you won't run out?

yes

12. Do you find it difficult to imagine life without smoking?

yes

13. Do you choose only activities and entertainments such that you can smoke during them?

Yes

14. Do you prefer, seek out, or feel more comfortable in the company of smokers?

Yes

15. Do you inwardly despise or feel ashamed of yourself because of your smoking?

Yes

16. Do you ever find yourself lighting up without having consciously decided to?

Yes

17. Has your smoking caused trouble at home or in a relationship?

Yes

18. Do you ever tell yourself that you can stop smoking whenever you want to?

Yes – at one time I believed that.

19. Have you ever felt that your life would be better if you didn't smoke?

Yes

20. Do you continue to smoke even though you are aware of the health hazards posed by smoking?

Yes

If you answered yes to one or two of these questions, there is a chance that you are addicted or are becoming addicted to nicotine. If you answered yes to three or more, you are probably already addicted to nicotine.*

---

* The Smokers Anonymous checklist of twenty questions is reprinted with permission of Smokers Anonymous World Services, 2118 Greenwich Street, San Francisco, CA 94123 (415) 922-8575.

I WANT TO
QUIT LIKE
MARK TRAIL DID

" But It's Not Easy to Quit..."

The comic strip hero Mark Trail quit smoking sometime in 1983. We were never told the exact date, but in mid-December he told his friends he had quit smoking his pipe. He went into no details, so we don't know if he suffered any withdrawal. He probably didn't, judging from the manner in which he told his friends. He just decided to quit, and he did.

That's how I want to quit. In fact, for more than twenty years that's how I thought I would quit. During all that time, I believed some day I'd just put out my cigarette and say, "That's it. No more. This just doesn't make sense." My expectations didn't seem unrealistic because I'd heard many people describe their quitting in those very words. Oh, most of them said they had to fight the craving for several days, but I knew I could do it if they did. A few said it was tough for a few weeks, and even that didn't seem to be impossible for me. *I can do that*, I thought. The prospect of being hit with an occasional intense craving even years later was okay too. As I began my first few attempts to quit, I was prepared for any of these things. I was willing to endure any of them because I "knew" from the experience of others that the worst symptoms are short-lived. Mine weren't, and I was unprepared.

Probably the most famous line on this subject is Mark Twain's: "It's easy to quit smoking; I've done it thousands of times." The fame of it rests on its popularity with smokers, who understand too well its truth. We've all quit thousands of times—most of those are bedtime promises, but some are actual periods of abstinence, followed by relapse. It is easy to quit—to promise ourselves or others. It's easy to last an hour or two, sometimes a day or week or two. What's difficult for most of us is to stay quit. Those of us who fail to stay abstinent are puzzled how others can do it. And they are often anxious to share their secret.

Over the years, I probably have been told a hundred sure-fire ways to quit smoking. A grapefruit diet was one of those secrets; cranberry juice was another. "Drink tremendous quantities of water," was the advice of a friend who quit painlessly. Keeping a journal for two weeks prior to quitting was supposed to help me understand my habit. It did help me understand when and why I smoke, but understanding didn't diminish my withdrawal symptoms when I quit. Two other well-meant pieces of advice that didn't help were "quit with a friend" and "go to a hypnotist." I combined the two, plus drank cranberry juice by the gallon. It was the worst experience I've had in all the times I've quit, probably because it was the longest.

Most advice given is simple; it seems to hinge on one food, item, or ritual. This doesn't mean some of these don't work for some people. Or is it possible that the person who quit smoking by eating fourteen grapefruit a day would have also quit by drinking water or cranberry juice or by going to an acupuncturist?

Some advice strikes me as silly. I was once told by a woman that she quit after she burned a hole in her favorite dress. I don't challenge the truth of what she told me, but I've never understood how such a thing could intervene in an addiction. Was she truly an addict or just a social smoker? This is the same friend who once had invited me over for coffee and when I lit my cigarette said, "I think I'll have a cigarette too. Now where are they?" She proceeded to look through cupboards and purses. Finally, she gestured slightly with an index finger as if to say, "Ah-hah" and went to the closet and withdrew a cigarette pack from her coat. "I knew they were here somewhere," she said, "because I remember picking them up when we left the party Friday night." The woman hadn't smoked for three days!

My children, too, give me advice on how to quit. They're concerned about me. They have been told in school about the shocking risks I'm taking; they've seen the frightening films.

My daughter has told me it's simple: all I have to do is say I won't smoke again no matter how bad it gets. "And you know, Mom, it would get better. Why don't you just say, 'I won't smoke even if it takes two years'?"

How many times have I heard the line, "If I can quit, anyone can quit." There are variations: "I just decided one day that enough is enough. I took that pack of cigarettes and threw it out the car window." Or, "I saw my best friend die of cancer, and I quit then and there." Directly or by implication, the speaker is telling us our failure to quit rests solely on us. I'm not sure which closing line I hate more, the one that goes, "It was tough, but I decided I was going to make it no matter what" or, "I tried to quit 477 times, but the last time was so easy. That was three years ago, and I've never missed them." The first tells me that I'm just not as strong as this person. The second makes me want to scream, "You mean it's not up to me, and I have to wait for a miracle?"

No one has a perfect understanding of why one person is successful and another is not. Or even why the same person might fail repeatedly and then succeed unexpectedly. The surgeon general's 1988 report defines *spontaneous remission* as the "intentional cessation of drug use, variously referred to as 'natural recovery,' 'maturing out,' 'burning out,' or 'self-quitting,' . . . Such quitting is sometimes reported to be due to 'will power' [sic] or 'just deciding to quit.'" The report cites the work of R. Stall and P. Biernacki in determining causes of spontaneous recovery (remission) from such addictions as alcohol, opioids, and tobacco. Their study, reported in the *International Journal of the Addictions,* identified several factors which may influence remission. Some of those were health concerns, social stigma, family, financial problems, accidents, and management of cravings. The surgeon general's report adds that ". . . persons most likely to quit use of tobacco and opioids without benefit of formal intervention do tend to have shorter histories of use and/or be at lower levels of dependence."

Have I smoked too long or too much? Is the level of my addiction so deep I can't pull myself out? I'm really not sure. I do know I've made repeated efforts to quit. The first time I tried, I was twenty-five and anxious to please my fiancé. I was quitting smoking, I told him by letter and by phone. And I quit for three weeks. My fiancé was overjoyed. I was overjoyed. I was also overconfident, and one day when offered a cigarette I took it, thinking it would be interesting to see what cigarettes taste like now. My relapse was immediate; by evening I had purchased and was smoking a pack of my old brand.

I stopped smoking again two years later when our daughter was born. This was more like a spontaneous cessation—I had no desire to smoke. Not for three days anyway, at which time the craving hit. At the end of two weeks, I caved in, but promised myself first that I wouldn't ever smoke in front of my baby. Soon I amended that to never smoking when I was nursing her. Finally, there were no amendments and no promises. The ensuing years were filled with similar promises, amendments, and failures.

There's a comfort for me in knowing my failures to quit are shared by others, but there's a sadness too. In some ways, it's been comforting to believe it was a lack of willpower because, if it was, then there's a possibility I would be stronger the next time. I could still have control and not be a victim of a disease. Each time I quit, I hope for greater control and more willpower. I listen eagerly to others as they share their secrets of success. "Don't drink coffee." "Don't eat meat." "Pray." I feel dishonest as I listen. As much as I want each new secret to work, I'm afraid it won't. Deep within my mind, I believe the secrets are really simplistic answers to a more complex problem. They are no more help to me than what my well-meaning son told me when he was eight: "It's easy to quit, Mom. Just don't buy any."

* * *

Sense and Nonsense

Nearly seven years have passed since my father's death. Illogical as it may seem, all four of us—his children—are still smoking, although one son has cut back to just a few cigarettes a week. A nonsmoker might think this is the height of foolishness or stupidity. Why would we choose to continue a habit that undeniably caused our father's death, a habit that likely will contribute to our own? It doesn't make sense.

I agree. Certainly, if my father's illness had been caused by eating grapes, I would have stopped eating grapes no matter how much I loved them. If the culprit were orange pop, I would never take another sip. If cedar siding, polyester clothing, or furniture wax had stimulated the cancer growth within my dad's body, I would by now have gone to any extreme to protect my loved ones and myself. It would be the intelligent thing to do, the right thing. Why then each day do I light thirty to forty cigarettes and expose my family, friends, and myself to the recognized dangers of smoking?

When I think about my smoking in a detached, logical, intelligent manner, I am confused and ashamed. I find myself agreeing with those who have directly or indirectly told me I am selfish, weak, and ignorant. The agreement comes easily because it confirms the secret, ugly self-talk I've carried around in my head for as long as I can remember. These inner messages may spring from some vague, long-ago feelings of inadequacy, but they're fed by the realities of what I see as proof of my inadequacies today:

- How can I, a mother of an asthmatic child, think myself anything but selfish as I callously expose her to my secondhand smoke?

- I'm weak, I tell myself, as I watch other smokers quit. I meekly listen to their monotonous theme song: "If I can quit, anyone can." I envy them and, at the same time, resent them. My repeated efforts to quit smoking fail. Why are these other people successful? The only answer I have is, they are stronger than I.
- Even elementary-aged children know the risks of using tobacco products, yet I ignorantly puff along as though it doesn't threaten me. *Dumb! Dumb! Dumb!* I say to myself.

It may seem to others that we tobacco users ignore the media's public service announcements, our chronic coughs, and our loved ones' pleas to stop. We may appear to not understand the dangers. I know what they are, and still . . . I don't know. It's as though the fear I experience when faced with those dangers actually forces the thoughts from my mind and calms me. I'm not ignoring the dangers. Most of the time, I'm really not even aware of them. On one level, I understand; then my mind quickly moves to another level, one at which the painful words and meanings can be submerged and forgotten. This isn't stupidity; it's denial.

During a nicotine addiction conference, the presenter was discussing how life crises—loss of job, family or financial instability—rarely affect smokers' lives and, therefore, very few of them see their tobacco use as an addiction. A member of the audience interrupted saying, "Oh, they have life crises, but the crisis is usually a fatal disease. By that time, it's too late." Unfortunately, all too true. I often have heard or read the words of a dying cancer patient who wants to warn other smokers, to tell us to quit, and to share his or her hard-earned insights even though "it's too late for me." To date, denial has served my addiction well, so that I've either pretended I never read or heard the warnings or have convinced myself that it won't happen to me.

The same denial said to be common for other addicts is at work in my life. My coughs I call colds ("Well, a smoker can get colds too, you know," I've snarled at my husband). I'm comforted (and ashamed of that comfort) by nonsmokers' heart problems, emphysema, and cancer. There's a parallel comfort for me when I hear of smokers who live into their eighties and nineties. I insist that smoking calms and relaxes me, when in fact I know that my physical and emotional dependency on nicotine creates most of the stress. I deny the dangers of secondhand (passive) smoking and declare my habit to be a personal choice.

Choice. That's a laugh. Within each day I make dozens—perhaps hundreds—of large and small choices. What to wear. What to have for breakfast. Or will I even eat breakfast? Dinner plans. Notes and last-minute directions to the children. Do the dishes or let them wait until later? As I move through the day, I have the power to decide which project to tackle first and which to forget entirely. As a writer, I choose one word or phrase over others. From morning until bedtime, I pick and choose. I look at options and decide.

One thing I don't decide, however, is whether to smoke. For me, a forty-seven-year-old woman, that decision was made nearly thirty years ago by a first-year college student. And even she wasn't intending to make a lifelong decision; she was just going to try one cigarette. And then maybe just one more. Another, and then another, and at some point, she lost her power to choose. She had become addicted, still believing she chose to smoke and denying the power and impact of nicotine in her life.

Belief in my power to choose, and denial of how totally nicotine has stripped me of that power, are my two greatest enemies. Many of us smokers continue to feed our minds a steady diet of negative self-talk: *If I cared about my family, I'd quit. This is so dumb. I'm so weak. What's wrong with me?* Ironically, the pain of such thinking creates the urge, the craving to smoke because our minds and bodies have learned to deal with discomfort and unpleasantness by using nicotine.

More unpleasant messages come from society at large,

which repeats out loud the same secret, ugly things we say to ourselves: "You're killing yourself." "You can quit if you really decide to." "Think of your family." "It doesn't make sense." Here, too, nicotine serves to quiet the voices, to diminish the guilt, and to create an invisible barrier between ourselves and the accusations.

"It doesn't make sense" is an opinion voiced by smokers and nonsmokers alike. And we're right, smoking and other tobacco use don't make sense—if we insist on emphasizing tobacco use as a matter of choice. Then we probably will continue to use words like *cessation* rather than *recovery*, *stupidity* rather than *denial*. And those of us who are addicted will seemingly ignore the physical and emotional symptoms of our disease. We will continue to use tobacco, believing ourselves weak. We will continue to disappoint our loved ones and shock medical professionals who expect us to act like nonaddicts by not smoking when they tell us not to. We will shell out billions of dollars, mostly for tobacco, but also for answers in the form of cessation programs, acupuncture, hypnosis, therapy, and quick-quit gimmicks advertised in the media.

If the message remains unchanged—that tobacco use is a habit, that users *choose* to ingest tobacco, that anyone can quit with a little willpower—then most of us will remain trapped, and young people will continue to ignorantly experiment with a drug they believe to be safe. And this, sadly, makes perfect sense.

* * *

"You're All Alike!"

If addiction is, as many people suggest, a progressive disease, it is understandable why it may be easier to quit earlier in the addictive process. That is, it might be easier to quit *if* the young addict attempts to quit. Many of us smokers don't try to quit until we're in our thirties and forties, after we begin to experience or fear a decline in our health. The casual manner with which we began smoking ("It only hurts old people") no longer feels so safe. Although not yet old, we've begun to see how smoking affects our chances of growing old. We regret the decision made by our younger selves, and we want to salvage as much time as possible. When we quit and fail repeatedly, we begin to have a vague sense of something being wrong. Others have quit. Why can't we? Are we just weak? Or are we more dependent on nicotine than those who are able to quit?

This is another area of nicotine addiction that researchers are examining. They are trying to determine the characteristics of hard-core smokers. Are we more compulsive in all areas of our lives? Are we more likely to be addicted to other drugs as well? Do these smokers share specific emotional or physical characteristics? Learning the answers to such questions may be of future use in the treatment of nicotine addiction, but the inconclusive data available today is of little help to those of us who haven't been able to quit.

Many cessation programs help smokers identify the reasons for their addiction—the "why," as one program calls it. Most people want to know what kind of smoker they are. It's comforting to have labels to put on our behavior. We want to understand it in hopes of conquering it.

Such programs are effective tools for many smokers. Why not for everyone? In a recent class I attended, eight people registered. Three attended all four sessions, two attended three sessions, two attended two, and the other didn't return after the first session. (I asked for permission from class members to attend without trying to quit although I did quit for six days.) Two of the women stopped smoking after the first night's session. Another did by the second session. A fourth woman quit for several days, but resumed smoking the day she was laid off from her job. The only man who attended quit the morning of the third session. I called them two months after our last session.

Three of the original eight members had not returned to smoking. They all agreed they had to occasionally fight craving. One described struggling with rationalization: *Well, I could probably smoke two or three cigarettes and still be all right.* Or, *Even if I start smoking again, I wouldn't be so bad because I know now that I can quit.* Another said she thought social situations had been the most difficult for her. They all mentioned social situations as prompting the urge to smoke.

Most of those who were unable to quit cited stress as the reason. Were these people under more stress? Or were they more susceptible to stress? Are they more dependent on nicotine as a manager of their emotions? Most of these people seemed to feel it was their fault they had failed. There was some guilt expressed, and great disappointment. "I failed again," one woman said, "but why did I think it could be any different this time?"

The question of fault and the sense of guilt haunt all of us who fail to quit. There's no way to measure our determination to quit. We believe we want to succeed as much as those who do, but are we deluding ourselves? Are we not as dedicated after all? Are we reserving conditions on quitting, such as how much interruption of our lives we'll tolerate? Is it us, or are there different levels of addiction? Do some people manage to quit more easily than we because we use nicotine in different ways, for different reasons?

Many smokers I've talked to are convinced that no one could have wanted to quit more than they did. I believe I've been as determined as anyone. If we do use our drug differently or for different reasons, perhaps what's needed are more flexible approaches, more alternatives for treating the different kinds or levels of addiction. If we are sincere in our attempts to quit, perhaps new approaches based on a recognition of the variety and complexity of nicotine abuse patterns will give us, the persistent failures, hope for recovery too.

* * *

Doctor, Doctor!

He's an excellent doctor, and I turned to him for help, for his expertise in dealing with my addiction. I used the word *addiction* when I explained to him my pains, my morbid fears, the stiffness throughout my body.

"I really think it's withdrawal from nicotine," I told him, "because I've been having these problems only since I stopped smoking seven months ago."

"It takes some people more time to get over it," he explained. "Just be sure you don't go back to it. You said your father died of lung cancer? Well, I just saw a woman about your age . . . " He looked at my records lying on the desk. "Yes, exactly your age. Forty. And she has the cancer your dad had—oat-cell cancer. I'm sure she'd do anything to go back to a time before she had it, and I'm just as sure she'd be able to quit smoking then."

"How?" I asked him. "I know these things. I know all the things that can happen to me, and here I am—not smoking and miserable. Not smoking and crazy, depressed, and aching all over. What can be done for my withdrawal so I don't go back to smoking? I don't want to smoke again. I hate it. But I'm afraid I'm going to if my health doesn't get better . . . if my life doesn't get better."

"You just have to fight it. I've never smoked, so I'm not sure what you're feeling like, but I know it's a strong habit. You wouldn't believe it but just the other day there was a patient in the hospital who lit a cigarette while receiving oxygen. I can't believe he did it. He knew the oxygen could explode. It just doesn't make sense."

Yes, he's a wonderful doctor—I would recommend him to anyone. As an oncologist (a cancer specialist), he's highly respected, but he had nothing to offer me that day.

I left his office as shaky and miserable as when I'd come in.

Perhaps even more so, because now I was sure nothing could be done to help me get through what I was calling my "dry drunk." Maybe I really was crazy, I thought, as I wandered to my car. After all, this brilliant physician couldn't understand why I'd even consider returning to smoking or why that patient in the hospital had insisted on smoking. And I thought that made perfect sense. What confused me was the doctor's attitude. Why would anyone expect an addict not to behave like one?

The lack of understanding between smokers and nonsmokers usually can be explained by one or more of the common myths about smoking.

- *Cigarettes taste awful, but smokers like the taste.*

Many nonsmokers have tried smoking once or twice and remember the disagreeable taste. After smoking regularly for some time, most cigarette users no longer experience that unpleasantness. Either their taste buds are numbed, or their brains have been conditioned to disregard the taste in order to better accommodate their addiction. Of course, some tobacco users do actually enjoy the flavor of tobacco from the very start and select one brand over another for its taste. But I don't think that's the real reason for continued use any more than an appreciation of fine wines explains an alcoholic's drinking patterns.

- *If the cost of tobacco products were considerably higher, everyone would quit.*

A leap of 400 or 500 percent would probably cause a substantial number of smokers to cut down or quit—at least for a time. Hard-core addicts, and especially those who could afford it, would continue smoking. An addiction is protected at all costs, and it's common for addicts to cut back on other expenses—even essentials—to accommodate the cost of the drug. A positive aspect of higher tobacco costs, though, would be its potential use as an intervention and prevention tool. If the addict continued using tobacco in the face of family members' clear deprivation, the cost factor could become a means of helping him or her face the reality of the addiction. High cost might also prevent some young people from experimentation with the drug.

- *Smokers are selfish, insensitive people.*

Smokers are just people and no different from nonusers in their potential for either selfishness or empathy. An addiction, however, is cruel and deceitful; under its power, a person who is normally caring and empathetic can be selfish and insensitive. Driven by craving, a smoker is likely to respond to smoking restrictions, whether imposed by etiquette or law, with denial messages such as the following: "No one will notice." "There's no reason smoking shouldn't be allowed here." "I bet if I light up, a dozen other people will too."

- *Better education about health risks can bring about a tobacco-free society.*

First of all, education has thus far proved to be most effective as a *deterrent* to drug use. Because of their denial, most addicts aren't likely to respond to "the facts" no matter how well they are presented. Those wishing to discourage youth from tobacco use should gear their educational messages to immediacy. Health or death risks discourage many young people from experimentation with drugs, but usually only if the risk is imminent. They may know or have heard of people their age dying from overdose of crack or heroin. But tobacco doesn't threaten most of them, because it doesn't threaten them now. From their perspective, tobacco kills "old" people. In the face of the most dire predictions, they experiment with tobacco, believing themselves safe. Recognizing this, many health groups are emphasizing the *immediate* risks of tobacco use for young people — decreased physical ability, cost, smell, and social stigma.

- *We can legislate a tobacco-free society.*

Legislation, like the cost factor, is probably most effective as an intervention or prevention tool. Increasingly, smoking is being prohibited. Government buildings, hospitals, restaurants, and many other facilities have gradually gone from allowing smoking virtually everywhere to setting severe limits. An increasing number of facilities — particularly health care institutions — have become totally smoke-free. The federal government has given impetus to this movement by requiring health warning labels on tobacco and prohibiting smoking on commercial airline flights of less than two hours.

Legislation leading to prohibition would probably be no more effective than our earlier attempt in the 1920s with alcohol — and for the same reason: an addict who is not recovering will use his or her drug and will get that drug no matter what the cost or inconvenience.

- *Smokers can improve both their health and their chances of quitting if they learn to smoke lighter or fewer cigarettes.*

Our bodies and brains function now with a demand for a certain level of nicotine. Even when we switch to a lighter cigarette, we run the risk of unknowingly changing our smoking strategy in order to get more nicotine. We might select a brand touted to be less dangerous, but then begin buying them in longer lengths. Or we might start smoking faster, inhaling more deeply, or covering the airholes in the filter to achieve greater absorption of nicotine in the lungs. Despite our best intentions, many of us end up smoking more cigarettes. Noticing this, we deny the danger by telling ourselves that at least the cigarettes have less tar and nicotine.

Also, it's more difficult today to know if we really are smoking a lighter brand of cigarette. For a time, the Federal Trade Commission published the nicotine and tar levels of every major brand of cigarette. According to Dolly D. Gahagan, author of *Switch Down and Quit*, the tar and nicotine levels of some cigarettes increased after the FTC stopped publishing those figures.

* * *

Withdrawal

Other smokers, when they realized I was interested in the subject of smoking, often began listing the symptoms they had during an unsuccessful attempt to quit. Many of these people were strangers, but they talked to me like old friends when they saw my sympathy, understanding, and belief. For many, it seemed a relief to find a willing listener.

Even some who had never tried to quit had stories to tell of friends. One man with whom I shared an ashtray in the lobby of a summer resort wrote down his name and phone number and urged me to call him about his friend who had quit smoking two years earlier. "She's had a total personality change," he told me. "It's unbelievable. She used to be outgoing, the life of the party. Now, she's quiet and never goes out. She's a recluse."

The primary reason—maybe the only reason—we fail to quit smoking is difficulty coping with symptoms related to the physical and psychological withdrawal from nicotine. These symptoms are as varied and far-ranging as the physical and psychological causes of smoking. It appears all of us do not experience the same symptoms, and although two smokers may have the same symptom—anger or depression or hunger, for example—the degree or severity can vary so much that their experiences are entirely different.

Most people who successfully quit smoking have, at the very least, some discomforts and cravings for a period of time. For these people, the symptoms gradually decrease in intensity, and by somewhere between the second and fourth week the worst has passed. Some people who have quit smoking say they did not feel they were truly free of the withdrawal symptoms until after the third month. A few say it was six months until they felt noticeably better. Information given to people trying to quit in more formal programs supports these general time lines. For some of us, this information is discouraging because our experiences with withdrawal do not even remotely come close to those of the people who are successful.

I wonder if this information is based only on the perceptions of people who have been able to quit, which means it doesn't reflect unsuccessful quitters' experiences. It may be, too, that others assume our withdrawal to be the same as those who are successful and that sheer motivation determines success or failure. It's difficult to know intuitively if our experiences are the same as, or different from, those of successful quitters. I would guess that others who fail are like me: They wonder if they just can't handle the stress of withdrawal as well as those who succeed. In accepting the reality of my addiction, I have to accept the deceptiveness of it. Clinging to the idea that my withdrawal pain is special, worse than that of others, may be another way to give myself permission to continue using nicotine.

My thinking runs back and forth between trusting my senses and suspecting my denial. I, like others, usually conclude that my senses are correct—I *am* motivated to rid myself of smoking and *have* tried as hard as I know how. Perhaps I've worked too much at finding the *right* way to quit or trying to understand why I fail. It may be that quitting smoking is not something like learning how to hang wallpaper, where it can be easy or difficult depending on how you approach it. Possibly it's more like childbearing—the mechanics are the same for every woman, but there's no explaining why one delivers in an hour and another is in labor for a day and a half.

The following list contains many of the withdrawal symptoms I've read about, experienced, or been told about by other smokers. This list is not research-based, which means it's possible some of these are symptoms of something else but were reported to me as occurring during withdrawal and disappearing with the resumption of smoking.

At first, I had decided not to include this list and to just state that anything occurring during abstinence might be due to withdrawal and that it should be checked out with a doctor. And then I remembered my experiences and state of mind when not smoking. It seemed for a time I was constantly going to this or that doctor for this or that complaint. As I think of it now, most physicians have little experience treating withdrawal, partly because we are reluctant to consult a doctor with early symptoms, and most probably we relapse before those symptoms get so severe. For a time, I checked out every book and article on quitting smoking and chemical dependency I could find. I skimmed through them, hoping to find my symptoms clearly identified as withdrawal. Depression was mentioned for other drugs but not for nicotine. Little was mentioned about nicotine withdrawal at all and its absence fed my secret fear that I really was crazy. More than anything, this list gives substance to what I've long suspected and now truly believe: I'm not crazy; I'm an addict.

- irritability
- anger/rage
- insomnia/wakefulness
- depression
- unprompted crying
- dreams of smoking
- anxiety
- health fears
- morbidity
- fatigue
- craving
- hunger/food binges
- increased intake of alcohol or other drugs
- cough and other cold symptoms
- cramping of arms and legs
- tightness in chest
- gastrointestinal upset (stomach pains, diarrhea, constipation)

- rashes/tender skin
- disorientation
- weight gain or loss
- mourning
- rationalization/fantasy ("I could be just a social smoker")
- inability to concentrate
- lightheadedness/dizziness
- sense of detachment from others/ emotional coldness
- forgetfulness

There are other vague complaints, such as a sense of incompleteness or of losing a sense of self. Some of us experience guilt, which is not surprising since many of us have used smoking to avoid consequences and responsibility for mistakes and hurting others. Some people say they aren't able to accomplish as much as they did when they were smoking. And it is possible that their disorientation and initial loss of concentration powers do temporarily reduce productivity. But for many, what has really changed is their *illusion* of accomplishment. As one woman said, "When I'm smoking— even if I'm doing nothing else—I feel as though I'm getting something done, as though I'm busy."

Please note, though, that extreme symptoms, whether depression, significant weight loss or gain, anger, or physical pain aren't necessarily symptoms of withdrawal and may be signs of other ailments. The possibility of an unrelated illness should be explored with a doctor.

It's sometimes difficult for us to hear about others' easy quitting stories, especially if we're in the early abstinence stage and somewhat angry anyway. Sometimes our anger is justifiable. One woman I talked to told of her anger toward her husband when they quit smoking together. He quit with no trouble, she said, but she suffered with severe withdrawal problems from the very beginning.

"He keeps telling me, 'You just have to make up your mind

to do it. Then there's nothing to it.' But you know," she told me, "I'm wondering if it's easier for him because he took up chewing tobacco when he quit smoking."

* * *

Cold Turkey

For most of my adult life, I thought I had beaten the odds. Despite having been raised in an alcoholic family, I was not an alcoholic, nor was I addicted to any other drug. What difficulties I did have were attributed to what is now commonly called the "adult children of alcoholics syndrome"—an assortment of issues such as low self-esteem, shame, fear of abandonment, perfectionism, and anger.

Never—ever—did I consider my cigarette smoking to be an addictive behavior. My many failures in attempting to quit, I saw as just that—failures, the feeble efforts of a weak-willed person. Then, in 1982, my opinion was changed forever. On February 5, less than one month after my father's death and one week before my fortieth birthday, I stopped smoking and resolved to never smoke again.

Prior to this, I had quit dozens of times for a few days, five times for three or four weeks, and of course thousands of times upon going to bed when I had promised myself I would quit the next day. Quitting was always difficult. The sheer act of willpower, of constantly resisting the urge to smoke, was exhausting, but I was proud of how strong I could be as I "white-knuckled" it through the cravings. Worse than the cravings for me, however, was the depression. I would become gradually sadder and sadder until I was virtually immobilized. The sadness disappeared each time I resumed smoking.

Even before Dad became ill, I had decided to quit smoking one last time, and I wanted to quit before I was forty. This time I decided to do it right and get some help, so I called a psychologist who had helped other smokers quit through the use of hypnotism. I explained to him my fears of becoming depressed again. He told me not to worry, that his "little trick," as he called it, would help me avoid the sadness.

He performed his trick. I paid him ninety dollars and went home. At the end of a week, I was a useless lump. My emotional range was despair to rage. Part of my rage centered on the psychologist, his patronizing attitude, and the fact I'd paid him all that money and felt no better than the times I'd quit by myself.

With the emotional distance that time has given me, I'm now able to see how easily I'd set myself up for disappointment. I'd wanted an easy answer, a less painful way to quit smoking. I had really expected to be "cured." Today, I can even see the humor of those expectations. When I failed to be cured of my habit, I assumed the hypnotism had somehow failed to take. I blamed my poor hearing and the fact that, when I was being hypnotized, I'd been sitting next to a window open to the noise of city traffic. Still believing a cure to be possible, I meekly returned to the psychologist and huddled down into the same chair next to the same window. But this time I tried to lean forward a little and listen more carefully to the magic words.

The magic, the cure, never happened. But believing what others told me—that it would get better—I fought the craving and endured the depression, minute by minute and day by day. Concentration became impossible; I couldn't write. By the end of the first month of abstinence, I had gained weight for the first time in my life (other than pregnancies). Even before the weight gain was noticeable, I had complained of feeling as though my skin was being stretched. When I crouched to pick up something from the floor, it felt as though a pair of socks were behind my knees. My skin was sore, as if the outer layer had been sanded away. On both sides of my neck, a numbness developed (similar to the effects of novocaine), and I was unable to turn my head very far.

The depression, weight gain, and stiff neck never let up in the months ahead. Then there was the insomnia, which wasn't true insomnia but rather a sudden wakefulness in the middle of the night. I would sit up with a start, as though I had overslept, and be so alert that I could not go back to sleep right away. This happened many times a night. My joints became painful. I stopped menstruating. My blood pressure, which had always been low to average (110/70 was normal for me), rose to a high of 150/96. I was angry (I stalked out of numerous stores because of imagined slights by clerks). I was sad (I wept several times a day because I thought my life was worthless) and awoke sobbing at night. I was morbid (I had wasted my life, and now, I thought, I had so little time left).

Although I described these symptoms to friends and family members as being withdrawal from cigarettes, I was just as skeptical as many of them were. What I really feared was, either I had developed some sort of fatal disease or I was going crazy, or both. I went to several doctors, either with specific symptoms or with the whole litany of symptoms, wanting to know if they thought these could be because I was not smoking. Their responses were just as varied as my complaints.

One doctor implied that I was there to get some sort of drug to lose weight and ended our visit by saying, "You smokers are just like alcoholics. You think if you quit, you should get a medal or a pat on the head." I broke down sobbing, and he left.

Another said my symptoms were probably stress-related and gave me a prescription for an antidepressant.

The most sensitive doctor I saw was the oncologist, who assured me that my higher blood pressure was due to the weight gain, not to quitting smoking. He encouraged my attempt to quit. He asked me what three things I would want to deal with or be rid of. The answer was easy: the depression, the stiff neck, and the continual weight gain. He wrote a prescription for a tranquilizer, and we made an appointment for me to come in again in two weeks. "I don't know what's causing this," he said, "but whatever you do, don't go back to smoking. You have to fight it."

Two days later I bought a package of cigarettes and cancelled the appointment. The pack was set up on the shelf where cigarettes had always been kept. I told myself I'd set a date, and if I didn't feel at all better by that time I would begin smoking again.

Some people would say that buying the cigarettes was the beginning of the end of my abstinence, and maybe they're right. I do know I didn't want to smoke and I didn't crave them. I just wanted to feel better, to be free of the sadness and numbness. I wanted to feel physically and emotionally healthy, and ironically the cigarettes seemed to be my only chance.

In a phone conversation with a close friend, I said that there was always the possibility that none of my problems had anything to do with not smoking. If that were true, then instead of being a depressed, overweight person, I'd be a depressed, overweight person who happened to be a smoker.

One morning, a week after I'd bought the cigarettes, my husband was leaving for work. I kissed him. He told me he hoped I'd have a nice day, and tears welled up in my eyes as they so often did. "Honey," he said, "you know there are worse things than dying young, and one of them is living like you are right now." I agreed and told him I'd already decided to go back to smoking in the hopes that things would be better. He looked so sad as he left; I felt worse for him than I did for myself.

The following Saturday, at three o'clock in the afternoon, I opened the pack of cigarettes, extracted a cigarette in my practiced fashion, and lit it. I took a long drag, pulled the smoke into my lungs, and exhaled. It had the same bitter, almost sour, taste as the first cigarette I'd smoked more than two decades earlier. Within seconds, a wave of lightheadedness hit me, just as it had when I was seventeen. Both of these sensations passed quickly, and I finished smoking the cigarette as though it had been minutes instead of months since I last smoked.

There was no immediate reaction other than guilt: I had failed—again. Then, barely fifteen minutes later, my neck felt better. Some of the numbness was gone; it seemed as though I could turn my head more easily. I dismissed it as being my imagination, as wishful thinking. Two hours later, I smoked another cigarette, and by that evening I knew I wasn't imagining it: the numbness was leaving my neck. My hopes soared that all my other problems would also disappear.

I resumed smoking on September 25, 1982—after nearly eight months of not smoking. Throughout that time, I had continued to gain weight—a total of forty pounds—but I began to lose as soon as I resumed smoking. Five pounds was gone after I'd smoked only three days; five more by the end of two weeks; and another ten by the end of seven weeks. The rest has stayed, but in one way I've returned to what is normal for me: my weight doesn't fluctuate greatly no matter how much or little I eat.

My husband, noting how little I was smoking, asked if I craved more. "No, that's the greatest part of the whole thing," I told him. "I don't need as many as I used to, and I'm still getting better."

Everything was getting better. No longer did my skin have the puffing up or stretching sensation. I could concentrate again. On October 12 I had minor outpatient surgery. My weight was nearly twenty pounds more than it had been eight months earlier, but my blood pressure had returned to normal: 110/70.

Normal. Our lives did return to normal. I was normal once again. But the relief, the joy, came with a terrible price tag—my freedom. I hadn't beaten the odds or escaped the legacy of family chemical dependency. For whatever reason, normalcy for me meant maintaining a steady level of nicotine in my body. On one hand, I was terrified of the intensity of my addiction, and, on the other hand, I was overjoyed to see how much "healthier" I was becoming each day.

By the following summer, the depression, the anger, the weepiness were gone. I was able to sleep through the night. The joint aches were much better. My optimism had returned. Life was good. I was smoking two packs a day.

*   *   *

INTERLUDE:
THE MECHANICS
OF ADDICTION

BY ANY OTHER NAME

Some people argue that we have become too eager to slap the label "addiction" on too many behaviors. What once was a term used only for dependence on alcohol and certain illegal drugs is now applied to dependence on prescription drugs, compulsive sexual behavior, gambling, overeating, anorexia, excessive spending and shopping, and now—of all things—nicotine.

The Symptoms Are Not the Disease

Some confusion might be due to our emphasis on the symptoms of alcoholism or of addiction to what are often labeled "hard-core drugs." These produce dramatic and predictable behaviors which have impact on people close to the addict and even on society at large. Innocent people are killed by addicts who drive under the influence of these drugs. Their overdoses often make headline news. The loss of control brought on by their disease affects the crime rate. They are more likely than nonusers to lose jobs, family, and friends. And, of course, the most familiar symptoms of the abuse of these drugs—the unkempt appearance, irregular gait, slurred speech—are often recognizable to the nonusing public. We can see these addictions. Because we can see them and because their effects are often so immediate and dramatic, it's easy to label them as serious addictions.

Yet, drunkenness and overdose are not the only criteria for defining addiction. They are obvious results of addiction to drugs which greatly alter the user's mood. Even marijuana, despite being illegal, seems to be taken less seriously than other drugs. If so, is this because its immediate effect on society is not as great as a drug like heroin?

Both marijuana and tobacco have been termed "gateway" drugs, which means using either of these may be the beginning, the gateway, to other, "more serious" drug use. By "more serious," I believe we are referring to the drugs that get more attention by causing greater problems for nonusers.

Of course, society *should* be concerned about the trafficking of illegal drugs. We are correct in our alarm over the proliferation of and increase in use of drugs such as heroin, cocaine, and crack. Still, this doesn't make it logical to tie the meaning of addiction only to its specific effects on society.

In other words, the symptoms of some addictions create very clear social problems, but this doesn't make addiction strictly a societal disease. It is also a personal, one-person-to-one-drug relationship.

I am an addict. My day-to-day functioning is dependent on using a drug. This drug keeps balance and control in my life. I don't function without it because everything about my past history with it tells me I can't. If this personal relationship were with alcohol or cocaine, my symptoms would be different. I couldn't as easily pass myself off as "normal." My family would be more certain to know the fear and shame associated with living with an addict. I would likely have to resort to more extreme measures to finance and conceal my use. My remorse would be greater because of the more obvious emotional damage to my family and friends. But the person-to-drug relationship – the heart of addiction – would be the same. It would be me and my drug getting through the day.

Drug of Choice

The word *choice* crops up often in discussions about tobacco use. The phrase *drug of choice* is commonly used in chemical dependency treatment circles. Yet *drug of choice* is not about choosing or deciding or logically selecting one drug over another. Whether alcohol, cocaine, heroin, or nicotine, *drug(s) of choice* is simply the primary chemical(s) to which a person has become addicted.

It's not known why a person becomes addicted to one drug or two drugs and not others. Why some people become addicted while others do not is an area of current research, but today there is no clear-cut answer. Because the odds of chemical dependency are greater if one's parents are chemically dependent, it seems likely that addictive traits are either learned or inherited, or both. In his book, *The Addictive Personality*, chemical dependency specialist Craig Nakken takes the position that it is relatively unimportant to examine one specific drug and the behaviors of a person addicted to that drug. Instead, he discusses the process of addiction as the steady, predictable development of an unhealthy "relationship with an object or event," whatever the object or event. He explains his position:

> Addiction has been viewed in a very limited way. The reason for this limited focus is because the treatment of addiction is a very young field. The development of treating addiction on any sizable scale started with the beginning of Alcoholics Anonymous in 1935, which concerned itself with a specific form of addiction—alcoholism. In contrast, most other fields of study start with a general knowledge of the subject and, as time goes on, the focus becomes more and more specific.
>
> Our knowledge about addiction started with a specific form of addiction and is now starting to be transferred to help people with other forms of addiction. Moreover, the addiction treatment field was not started by a group of professionals, but by people who suffered from one specific form of addiction. As more and more about the nature of addiction was learned from these pioneers, it was found that their principles of recovery were also useful to help people with other addictions. As more knowledge was shared, persons

with other forms of addictions started using these principles to recover. Thus came the start of Gamblers Anonymous, Narcotics Anonymous . . . and other Twelve Step self-help groups.

Presently, our field is learning again. We are starting to ask new questions and are finding answers.

Why do certain principles of recovery work so effectively for all of these seemingly different groups? The apparent reason is that the same illness is being treated: addiction.

Millions of us who use tobacco are accustomed to thinking of our use as a habit, something we've chosen to do that soothes and comforts. The people around us, the media, our entire society reinforce this perception of habit by accepting—sometimes even encouraging—the notion that tobacco relieves our tenseness, that we can quit or cut down by sheer willpower, and that we choose to start or continue our tobacco use. For many, perhaps most, of us this is not true. Tobacco relieves tension for the addict primarily because use of the drug ends the craving for that drug. Our quitting or cutting down is generally not permanent; willpower alone—although successful for some—usually ends in relapse.

Nicotine is our drug of choice, but we didn't choose it *as an addiction.* We innocently and ignorantly drifted into an addictive relationship with this drug. Although on the surface it may appear that nicotine addiction is far different from other chemical abuse, it really isn't. We use and abuse our substance in many of the same ways and for many of the same reasons as any other addict.

We aren't really discussing choice when we talk about drug of choice. We're talking about the drug that's number one in maintaining the deception that locks a person into immature problem solving. For some, it is alcohol. For others, it is prescription drugs, or cocaine, or heroin. For millions of us, it is nicotine.

Tolerance

Usually, early drug use is sporadic and in low doses. Although many people will drink excessively, even early on, it usually is due more to their inexperience with the cumulative delayed effect of alcohol than to a driving need for the drug. Whatever drug is used, the effect is generally very dramatic at first. But then as the body adapts to the drug, the effect with the same dosage is lessened. This is known as *tolerance.* In an addicted person, the reason for taking the drug is the effect. As the body's tolerance increases, the user—either knowingly or unknowingly—adjusts intake upward either by increasing the dosage or by frequency of use.

Tolerance occurs with nicotine in much the same way it does with other drugs. Our body's initial reactions to the poisonous effects of nicotine can include nausea, dizziness, and sometimes vomiting. These symptoms quickly disappear with repeated use because the body develops tolerance to the drug. A predictable cycle occurs from that point forward. The body develops further tolerance; dosage is increased. The new dosage is tolerated; a higher dosage yet is needed. This continues for most smokers to a point at which a minimum level of nicotine is maintained (with peaks following each use), which provides a sense of well-being. For most smokers, this requires at least a pack of cigarettes a day, and for many, two or more packs. Not smoking or stress will trigger the brain's need for nicotine, which results in a craving that is immediately removed by smoking. Even during sleep—an unstressful time for most people—the bloodstream has a steady level of nicotine, which is usually enough to allow a full night's sleep.

Discussion of number of cigarettes smoked can be confusing, because smokers unknowingly develop smoking strategies that increase nicotine intake. Smoking machines are used to rate and rank the tar and nicotine levels of specific brands, but smokers can adjust those levels by rate of inhalations (from four to fourteen drags per cigarette or more) and the depth of the inhalations.

Easy Answers

For most addicts, our relationship with a particular drug began in our teens or, at most, our early twenties. We probably had expectations of what and who we should be at that age, and if we had to condense those expectations into a one-word definition, that word was *adult*. We were in the process of shrugging off the ties to our families and trying to acquire the trappings of adulthood. Most of us who have older children can remember seeing those children visibly change from one day to the next as they deliberately set out to define themselves. The change may have been in clothes, hairstyle, or even in how they talked and carried themselves. Children in their teens often experiment in these ways, I think, in order to find the safety they've lost by cutting themselves off from their families. With less family control and guidance, they feel vulnerable and frightened.

For some of us, for whatever reason, the vulnerability and fear are assuaged by a specific drug. It brings that feeling of safety. For me it was a sense of balance, of being strong, confident, and in control. I ignorantly believed I had grown up. All the qualities I had lacked, now suddenly and miraculously seemed to be mine. I could *control* my fears and pain.

Psychiatrist M. Scott Peck, in *The Road Less Traveled*, says we too often forget that pain is a natural part of living, and that "since life poses an endless series of problems, life is always difficult and is full of pain as well as joy." The addict doesn't learn this lesson and learns, instead, to medicate and numb even the smallest emotional discomforts. It seems to me now that we lock ourselves into a sort of perpetual "teenagedom." That small block of time in which I should have learned coping skills to deal with life's inherent pains and problems has stretched into a lifetime of avoiding pain and disallowing myself such feelings as anger, disappointment, and fear. Ironically, while I thought I was maturing and becoming independent, I was really becoming dependent on something outside myself to take care of me, something that could "kiss it and make everything better."

An almost instant relief comes with the inhalation of cigarette smoke: within seven seconds the nicotine hits the brain. Smoking is a learned behavior, and we who became addicted to it are no different from the laboratory rats who learn to run elaborate mazes to earn the sought-after reward. The reward ingrains the behavior. If tobacco no longer contained nicotine, I would no longer light cigarette after cigarette, any more than a rodent would continue to run a senseless, meandering course if the reward weren't offered. And because I am addicted, I am likely to seek the same quick answers in another substance or behavior if deprived of nicotine.

It's no mystery why young people so easily succumb to the lure of nicotine. First of all, this is a time of experimentation for all of us. Very few forty year olds are tempted to try "just one," but teens and preteens are open to trying new things as acts of independence, risk taking, and sometimes defiance. Then, too, the same forty year old is not being encouraged by friends to experiment, while a young person is often pressured by peers. Finally, there is the vulnerability of young people at a stage in life filled with uncertainty. The emotional and sometimes physical distancing from parents is a necessary part of growing up, but with it comes the fearfulness of working without a net. Life no longer seems as safe and predictable. Yet this is exactly how they learn to trust their own problem-solving ability; this is how they mature. If drug use becomes a quick and easy answer to their inevitable fear and uncertainty, then young people become eternal children.

Maturation is stifled when discomfort is handled by using a mood-altering substance rather than by learning to trust inner resources and the support of others. At the slightest indication of a painful thought or situation, some of us learned the automatic response of seeking instant relief. And nicotine never fails. In seconds, we can feel the sweet calming of nicotine. Fears and worries seem to disappear. Peck puts it this way:

> Fearing the pain involved, almost all of us, to a greater or lesser degree, attempt to avoid problems. We procrastinate, hoping that they will go away. We ignore them, forget them, pretend they do not exist. We even take drugs to assist us in ignoring them, so that by deadening ourselves to the pain we can forget the problems that cause the pain. We attempt to skirt around problems rather than meet them head on. We attempt to get out of them rather than suffer through them.

Drug *dependency* means just that: we're dependent on something outside ourselves to give balance and meaning to our lives.

DENIAL

An addiction must be protected at any cost, and perhaps the greatest price most of us pay is sacrificing our honesty. We don't necessarily become outright liars; that's too obvious. We veil our dishonesty in half-truths and white lies, which is to say we use denial to conceal the reality of our addiction from ourselves and others.

An Answer for Everything

For years I've been at one of two stages—just getting a cold or just getting rid of one. At least that's what I tell my family and friends when they comment on my cough. And this is partially true. I probably do get colds and bronchitis more often now than years ago; the damage smoking has caused my lungs creates a perfect environment for the cold virus. I'm not lying exactly, but I'm not telling the truth. And I try to avoid telling anyone how concerned I am about the frequent colds, and the constant cough to clear my lungs.

My daughter's asthma is not brought on by cigarette smoke, I explain to anyone who seems critical of me on this point. She has viral asthma, I tell them, which means her lungs go into asthmatic spasms in response to viral infections, and naturally I don't smoke so much around her when she's having an attack. I don't tell them how much I do smoke, even when she's having breathing problems. I don't tell them that my smoking patterns were not different when we thought she might be allergic to cigarette smoke. I just say, "Smoking doesn't bring on her attacks."

Denial is essential to every addict. We couldn't blissfully engage in our addictions if we had to be feeling guilty or fearful every time we did. So we deny why we use, how we use, and how it affects us and the people around us.

Although inwardly we may feel powerless and wish we could quit, to the world we proclaim messages that imply we like it and choose to do it:

- "Smoking relaxes me."
- "I smoke to help maintain my weight."
- "It gives me something to do with my hands."
- "I only smoke when I'm with other smokers."

And from the smoker who tried to quit and relapsed:

- "I decided I wasn't feeling any better."
- "I just remembered how much I like to smoke."

"I Don't Really Smoke That Much"

We smokers also will frequently fool ourselves and those concerned about us into thinking we smoke less than we do. Most of us have claimed that many of our cigarettes burn down untouched in the ashtray, or that we only smoke them halfway down when, in fact, this rarely happens. We focus on the few times it does. This allows us the denial of how many cigarettes we really smoke and how completely we smoke them.

Many fellow smokers I've talked to have mentioned the necessity of buying cigarettes by the carton. Doing so allows us to deceive those around us as to how much we smoke and serves to help us forget how often we need a new pack. If we had to purchase cigarettes pack by pack (or worse yet, ask others to purchase them for us), it would be harder to conceal the amount from others and ourselves. Another concealing tactic I share with many other smokers is keeping ashtrays emptied. Somehow we delude ourselves into believing that, if our family or friends don't see the butts, we must not have smoked the cigarettes.

Perhaps one of our best denial tools is our willingness to buy into the "new and improved" myth in cigarette advertising. The introduction of the filter tip not only helped keep those little irritating bits of tobacco out of our mouths, it helped us distance ourselves from the nagging fear of what we were doing to our bodies. The advent of low-tar and low-nicotine cigarettes further engages the same denial. "I decided to give up cigarettes," one woman joked, "so now I smoke [a popular low-tar brand]."

Some cigarettes have small vent holes around the filter to diffuse the smoke before it enters the mouth, and they do deliver low levels of nicotine when tested by cigarette smoking machines. But because smokers' bodies and minds demand a certain accustomed level of nicotine, many smokers—either deliberately or unconsciously—block the vent holes as they drag off the cigarette, which of course increases substantially the amount of nicotine inhaled. Carrying this kind of denial to the extreme, at least one smoker that I know of selected a particular brand because of its low tar and nicotine ranking, but before smoking each one, crisply twisted off its filter tip.

Control

The belief we can control when, where, and how much we use is part of many a tobacco user's denial system. "I never smoke at work." "I don't smoke before breakfast." The message is clear: "I can't be an addict because I can control it." By seeming to control our addiction, we attempt to control the reactions of those around us. If others can be convinced we're not driven by a drug, then our use is okay. (This need to have others believe we are in control is, I believe, the reason many of us conceal our use.) The need to seem in control is indicative of the very addiction we're trying to deny. People who aren't addicted generally don't try to prove it and don't have to work so hard to convince others.

Our attempts to manage or control our nicotine use often drive us toward other compulsions or lock us into long-term withdrawal. Although our metabolism is changed by nicotine, the cases of extreme weight gain when quitting smoking are more likely due to compulsive eating or drinking—an attempt to find comfort and balance in another substance. It is a case of the eternal child being suddenly thrust into a grown-up world of pain, problems, and decisions.

Deprived of their drug without receiving treatment, addicts often will seek the same relief and chemical balance by using other drugs or by engaging in other compulsive behaviors, or both. This act of switching ties into the need for control. Craig Nakken says switching "helps create the illusion that the 'problem has been taken care of,' when in reality one dangerous relationship has been replaced with another. This buys time for the addict." Nakken uses the examples of an addict switching from speed and pot to drinking and how an "alcoholic who hasn't accepted his addictive personality may slowly develop an addictive relationship with food, putting on fifty or sixty pounds and remaining as emotionally isolated as when he was drinking."

The Healthy Smoker

We can also deny our addiction by finding comfort in our own and other smokers' apparent health. We all know many smokers, and most of them seem fairly healthy. Perhaps the health warnings are exaggerated, we think. Listening to all the diseases we're supposedly courting, one would think smokers would be expiring on the street left and right, like a scene from a movie about the Black Plague. But that's not happening. And hey! I feel good; I never felt better.

In the fall of 1988, I was given a good dose of "healthy smoker" denial when a radio talk show host made reference to a recent game involving our local baseball team. The host mentioned that one of my favorite players had hit a home run during a recent game, and after the player had loped around the bases, he ran straight into the exit ramp where he lit up a cigarette. Hearing this made me feel better about myself. When an athlete (a celebrity too) is able to compete on a professional level despite being a smoker, why should I worry?

Fatalism

Sometimes, denial pushes us into an unacceptable or impossible position. The denial of choice ("I think I'll quit on Christmas Day") forces us into a panic as the days leading up to Christmas evaporate at a speed-of-light pace. Some of us make a stab at quitting, but more likely one of our other denial strategies will save us that pain. Quite often, it is fatalism.

"I've smoked for thirty years. The damage is already done," we may tell anyone who asks. Or we combine fatalism with choice and control: "I decided not to quit now. What good would it do since my husband still smokes? I told him I'm going to quit when he does."

Or we might adopt a totally fatalistic philosophy of life:

"I'm going to just enjoy life as it comes. I could be hit by a truck or struck by lightning. There are no guarantees, you know, so I'm not going to get into the hassle of quitting. And besides, look at what happened to Joe down the street. Dead at thirty-seven, and he never smoked a cigarette in his life."

Rationalization

Rationalization is closely related to denial, but it is used by us addicts to deal with the issues that can't be denied. If someone confronts us with our inactivity, we maintain we're just more laid-back (or mellow or cerebral) than others. If we can't get through a movie or a wedding reception without smoking, we say we were bored or needed to get some air. When our denial system fails, we fall back on any of the hundreds of rationalizations at our disposal.

- "Smoking relaxes me."
- "I deserve one vice."
- "At least I'm not hurting anyone else."
- "I don't smoke as much as a lot of other people."
- "I'm not making my family go bankrupt with this habit."

I have even joked with my children about how lucky I am that birth weights are lowered by mothers' smoking. I probably couldn't have delivered any of them if their birth weights hadn't been significantly lowered, I've told them. Two of them weighed eight and one-half pounds and the other was over nine pounds.

The drug becomes the center of the addict's existence. Slowly, insidiously, it supplants decision-making powers, often without the addict being aware of it. This is why so many of us insist we're *choosing* to drink or smoke or use other drugs—it feels as though we are deliberately using the drug. Only when we attempt to quit using are we faced with the fact that we aren't our own people. Even then, the twisted thinking of addiction may convince us that we'll quit at a later date because (a) there's too much stress in our life right now, (b) our family didn't support us enough this time, or (c) we want to finish the pack or the bottle or the prescription first. Or we use any of the endless rationalizations which enable us to think we're still in control.

It's relatively easy for the addict to believe denial statements because they're essentially based in truth. Joe down the street did die at thirty-seven. Some celebrities do smoke. I do intend to quit on such and such a date.

What makes these statements even more dangerous is that the people around us also either believe them or choose not to challenge them. Their belief or acceptance of our denial enables us to blithely puff away. The denial system of any addict can be cut away by loved ones, but only after those friends and family members confront and rid themselves of their enabling of the addiction. It may be that until that time, or until a life crisis destroys our denial system, we will continue to be driven by this emotional, physical, and spiritual disease.

ENABLING

As humans we strive for order and balance. When our lives are chaotic, we work to restore equilibrium. Families, or anyone living with people addicted to drugs, especially those that cause extreme mood swings, become marked by the addict's unpredictable, erratic behavior. The unwritten rules of effective role formation and interaction are thrown out by the addiction. Common sense is replaced by nonsense. There is no equality among family members; the addiction becomes an additional member and demands all the power, all the money, all the decisions. Individual identities are lost in the turmoil.

To the nonaddicted members, it appears that the addict and the addiction are one and the same, and each person seeks to find meaning and balance in a contradictory and unbalanced relationship. A sense of being unacceptable and unloved is often engendered by the belief that the addict is choosing his or her behavior. Spoken or unspoken, spouse and children live with the conviction: "If you really loved me, you'd quit."

Buying into the Disease

One of the easiest ways for those close to the addict to make sense of the addiction is to buy into the addict's denial system. They begin to distrust their own sense of reality and to accept their lives as normal. In my relationship with my father, I was well into my thirties before I realized some people put the bottle away after mixing a drink, or that other farmers were probably not having a couple double shots of bourbon before their morning or lunchtime coffee, or both. My family had come to view this kind of behavior as normal because its predictability gave us the illusion of safety. For years we accepted the denial messages of his addiction: "I only had a couple." "I never get any help around here." "I'll be home for lunch." "I bought that bottle almost a month ago."

Stripped of a sense of balance in family relationships, members begin to live a teeter-totter existence. New identities evolve that can more easily accommodate the addiction and make sense of it. Self-worth as an inward balance becomes distorted into an outward attempt to keep the addict happy. The need for personal power is translated into attempts to control the addict. As family members struggle to find more balance and meaning in their existence, they increasingly accept and become perpetuators of the denial system. They lie to the outside world and to each other: "He has the flu." "She has a headache and is lying down." "I don't believe we received that bill in the mail." They *enable* the addict to continue his or her drug use while creating for themselves the illusion of power and control.

My father's disease became the property of us, his family, and we became obsessed with controlling and curing it because secretly we felt that we were causing it. Because we believed this, we tried harder to please and strived to give an impression of perfection to those outside the family.

The focus in a dysfunctional family is always outward—on the addict and the outside world. The learned coping skills emphasize management of someone else, rather than developing independent living skills. Living this way is like owning a block of shares on the stock exchange. Early indicators are watched closely so decisions can be made. There are bull and bear markets—times for daring and times for caution—but it all depends on some mysterious outside force over which a shareholder has no control.

"How's Dad doing?" I'd always ask my mother on my trips home from college.

"He's been better lately," she would tell me. I could let my guard down a little. We worked for years to control the uncontrollable. We chose our words carefully, avoiding subjects we knew to be dangerous. During any conversation with my father, my mind would be whirling like a computer doing an association search: would this answer remind him of this dreaded subject, or would this word remind him of that person? Of course, the one subject we never allowed was his drinking. We believed his denial, and the denial said he *chose* to drink.

Protecting Illusions

Enabling often becomes a means for families to cope with other addictive behaviors too. The mother of an anorexic isn't uncaring when she seems to allow the steady decline of her child. She may have nagged and threatened her daughter about not eating and weight loss for months, only to be rewarded with unpredictable personality changes and anger.

"I like how I look!" the daughter screams in denial. And faced with her loss of power and the increasing chaos in the family, the mother acquiesces and accepts the denial—she becomes an enabler.

On another occasion, the mother might express concern again by asking if the daughter ate her lunch at school. As the girl lies, the mother believes her because to challenge her would mean facing powerlessness. A dysfunctional pattern of denial and enabling begins, and it probably would have developed if the girl had been addicted to alcohol or another drug or to an obsessive behavior like gambling or sex.

What is so frightening about denial and the enabling it fosters is that everyone involved believes it. We *really* believe it. Our minds accept the unbelievable, the abnormal, because to do otherwise would unearth the chaos. The illusion of balance and control is so essential to our minds, that we will make sense out of nonsense.

In recent months, two of my children have begun nagging again about my smoking. I have told them I'm going to quit as soon as this book is done, and that silenced them. But why should it? First of all, why don't they challenge my contention that I can't write when I'm quitting? And why don't they ask me how in the world do I think I'm going to quit when I'm finished with the book when I've never been able to before? They haven't asked these things and they won't because such questions would contradict and threaten the balance and predictability of our family. To ask might necessitate looking honestly at my addiction. It would force them to admit I'm not in control and—worse yet—that *they're* not in control of my behavior. As it is, they've nagged me, and I've told them I'm going to control this on such and such a date. They've retained their illusion of control: they've made me promise to quit smoking.

Sometimes enabling families of smokers give outright permission: "Jack enjoys his pipe so much." "She was a smoker when we got married, and I don't think I have the right to change her now." Or they mouth the smoker's denial statements: "She's just smoking a low-tar, low-nicotine now."

"He smokes only four cigars a day." "He feels so much better since he quit smoking and started chewing tobacco." Their enabling buys into the denial system, and this creates a false sense of balance and harmony. It is false because what it does is allow the tobacco user to continue the addiction unthreatened and uninterrupted. Genuine concern will prompt them to make noises from time to time, but by and large they won't challenge the twisted logic that condones inhaling (or chewing) a poisonous substance.

An Enabling Society

Society as a whole can also be an enabler of tobacco use. Enabling occurs in a culture or community for the same reasons it occurs in a family—belief in the addicts' denial system and the need to make sense of unreasonable behavior. Nearly one-fifth of the American population are smokers. Add to that the millions of family members, and you have a large proportion of society denying or enabling the use of tobacco, or both.

We who have not been able to quit our tobacco use have stirred up emotional questions in our society. Why do some people fail in their attempts? Why don't others try to quit? Our behavior, when confronted with the health hazards in smoking and the benefits in quitting, makes no sense. And like the family that must make sense of illogical behavior, a society, too, can accept the denial statements of the addict: "I don't want to quit." "I enjoy smoking." "I choose to smoke." Some of society's beliefs and myths perpetuate illogical enabling behavior:

- Smokers choose to smoke.
- Smoking is a habit.
- Our power to convince smokers to quit lies in information and education.
- Anyone can quit.

- Smokers will quit when they're ready.
- Higher costs of tobacco will persuade smokers to quit.
- Once smokers are abstinent for a few days (weeks, months), they lose the desire to smoke.
- We can legislate a nonsmoking society.

All of these statements are based on the illusion of society's (including government agencies, health organizations, and cessation programs) control and power. A culture can be like the family whose dysfunctional logic locks individual members into a system that preserves an illusion by not really ever challenging the addict's denial system. This is frightening because there is probably nothing harder to abandon than an illusion that has finally made sense of craziness—especially an illusion that promises power and control.

A WAY OF LIFE

A WAY OF LIFE

The Grocery List

I spend so much time at the grocery store, that once when I'd failed to make my daily trip to the store, the grocer sent me a get-well card. This is a slight exaggeration, of course, but it does seem sometimes like all I do is handle groceries. I make grocery lists, go to the store, carry the groceries into the house, put the groceries away, cook the groceries, throw the paper containers into the garbage, and carry the garbage out to the curb. The sight of the ever-lengthening list on the kitchen counter fills me with dread of yet another trip to the store, and I try to make do and postpone it as long as possible.

One evening recently, I was hit by a sudden shortage of essentials. About to do dishes, I remembered we were out of dish soap. Oh, well, the laundry detergent did nicely.

My younger son decided to have a bowl of cereal. "We're out of milk," he announced from the refrigerator.

"Fix yourself a sandwich, if you're hungry," I suggested.

His face twisted into a grimace suitable for labeling poisons.

"Yuk," he said. "Aren't you going to the grocery store?"

"No, I don't think so. It's thirty below zero. I'm not about to run the car five blocks for some milk, and I'm certainly not going to walk. You can if you want to."

He declined my offer and decided to make cookies. "Where's the flour?" he asked from halfway inside the cupboard.

"I'm sorry. We're out of that too. I forgot. Why *don't* you have a sandwich?" He showed me that face again. Several other suggestions met either with his disapproval or the realization we were out of a needed item. No apples. Three black bananas that I had to use a spatula to pick up. No rolls. "Well, fix yourself a sandwich and stop complaining," I snarled at him after he made the Mr. Yuk face once too many times. I grabbed my cigarette case and ashtray and joined my husband in the living room where he was reading.

As I lit my cigarette and felt myself calming down, I suddenly realized I must have been smoking quite a bit that evening. I had opened this pack—the last of the carton—at four o'clock, and there was only one cigarette left.

I looked over at my husband, still so intent on his book. "You know," I said to him, "I really was snappy at Todd. I feel so bad. Guess I'll go up and get the groceries. We'll need milk in the morning anyway."

* * *

A Note from Mother

My perception of tobacco has changed so slowly I've hardly been aware of it. Only after I look back to where I once was do I see my progress. How I regard vending machines has been one of those gradual changes. At one time, I hardly took note of them. Then, as I became more convinced that nicotine was addictive and started monitoring my (and others') intake more closely, I began to notice these machines in a new light. They're everywhere, dispensing an assortment of food and candy and spitting out packages of cigarettes to anyone with a handful of quarters. Cigarettes cannot be legally sold to minors in most states, yet these machines are seemingly above the law as they indiscriminately provide kids with a drug that humans cannot legally sell them. I wonder how this can be.

I've intended to write letters to policy- and lawmakers and question the wisdom of allowing this, but I suppose they'll tell me (if they answer me at all) that the machines are intended to be a convenience for smokers. But why do smokers especially deserve this kind of convenience? Cigarettes are unquestionably linked to all sorts of "inconvenient" diseases, so for whose convenience is it to lean these contraptions against every available four-foot wall space?

This correspondence will likely never take place. I rarely write letters, to which neglected family members in far-off places will attest. So, instead, I just take note of the multiplication of these machines, and make insincere promises to try to do something about it—sometime.

A grocery store I went to recently had no vending machine. Perhaps it never had any, or it may have removed them to make way for a bank of computerized games blinking and babbling along one wall. Young people were gathered around one of them, watching a boy play a basketball game. This was one of the talking machines, and the crowd of children stood silently watching and listening as the voice described the game. They didn't notice me as I walked past them to get a carton of cigarettes from the adjoining wall rack and then hurried to the checkout counter.

I paid for it and was returning to my purse the few bills left me from my twenty when I noticed a young girl, maybe fourteen, behind me. She grasped a package of cigarettes in one hand and offered two one-dollar bills to the clerk with the other. I hesitated. *Here I am,* I thought, *buying cigarettes and thinking about questioning her right to buy them too.* But then that good-intentioned voice in my head, the one that's always telling me I should write and protest the wrongs I see, spoke up before I could stop it.

"You're not old enough to buy cigarettes, are you?" the voice asked.

The girl's eyes veiled over with a glare. She stiffened and pulled herself up straight. Her head moved slowly as if to find the source of this stupid voice. Her hand which held the money dropped the bills onto the counter and then reached into her pocket. Out it came holding a crumpled piece of paper. Her voice had a slow, singsongy rhythm and a tone reserved only for the very ignorant. "I have a note from my mother," she said. The voice within me was silenced.

* * *

Friendly Advice

"Do you know how much cigarettes cost?" she excitedly blurted out when I answered the phone.

I laughed. I thought she was joking.

"No, really. Do you know how much they cost?"

"Sure I do," I told her. "I've been buying them forever. Listen, can I call you back? I've got to run the kids to school so I can have the car."

The conversation is typical of a friendship that's spanned sixteen years. We both have families, and neither of us has the time, inclination, nor energy to devote to an orchid-like friendship requiring hothouse nurturing. We give snippets of time here and there, contentedly knowing the friendship will thrive with a minimum of care. We've never argued or hurt each other. We live ten miles from each other, but get together rarely. When we do, it's at one of our kitchen tables hunched over our coffee and cigarettes and talking like college roommates.

Most of our contact is by phone. Our calls at times have been an hour or more, but those have been rare troubled times. Usually the calls are brief. We've laughed about how brief most of them are. Often when I call her, she says, "Listen, I can't talk now. Can I call you back in a few minutes?"

I tell her that will be fine, and I go about my life. It might be two weeks before she calls back.

"I have company right now. I'll call you in the morning," I explain. And I might call her in the morning, or I might forget. If I forget, it's all right. The friendship is comfortable because there's no need to explain or apologize.

I called her recently. She couldn't talk, she said. "Are you going to be home tonight? I'll call you back then. I've got a meeting going on here," she told me.

"No," I said. "Tell them to go home." We laughed and agreed she'd call after dinner.

When she called the next week, it was to ask if I knew how much cigarettes cost.

She continued, "I'm serious. I mean out of a cigarette machine. I went to have coffee uptown and forgot my cigarettes, so I bought them out of a machine. Kid, I'll tell you, I just kept pumping quarters in until I didn't think I'd ever stop. Anyway, I don't think I've noticed how expensive they've gotten to be; I always buy the cartons with my groceries. It really made me stop and think, *What am I doing spending all this money?* It's scary! I don't know what to think or do."

For several years, cigarettes and smoking were a large part of our conversations. Much of our bonding had occurred during a stretch of time when we tried to quit smoking. During that period, our phone calls were long and daily. Even today, many years later, much of our honesty and trust in each other is rooted in that time when we struggled through withdrawal together. Each of us was fragile and vulnerable then. It was almost like we'd seen each other's devils, and we understood and were kind. Occasionally, we still confess we'd like to quit, but end up agreeing we'll never "go crazy" again.

Hearing her talk about the cost of cigarettes made me wonder if she was going to try again. A loving friend like me could encourage her. Perhaps a friend *should* encourage her.

"Well," I asked her, "are you going to try to quit?"

"No. Not now. But it really bothers me to see how much I'm spending. What am I going to do?"

"Don't buy them out of the machines anymore," I told her. "Keep buying them with the groceries if you don't want to know."

"Right. Thanks," she said with a laugh. "I'll call you tomorrow if you're home." She hung up.

* * *

Honeymoon

My husband and I had been married several years before I admitted to having fooled him. Until that time, he had believed I was not smoking at the time of our marriage. I had quit for three weeks in the fall before our wedding the following June, and when I started smoking again, I was sure that I'd be able to quit again sometime in the intervening eight months. He had been so pleased that I'd quit I hated to disappoint him with the bad news, so I didn't tell him. Two hundred miles separated us at the time which made it easier to conceal my smoking.

In May it occurred to me that I'd better stop smoking again soon, but with wedding details and all . . .

At 11 o'clock on the morning of June 22, 1968, my matron of honor and I were sitting at my family's kitchen table drinking coffee and smoking. Actually, we were drinking coffee, smoking, and attempting to attach fake nails to the chewed nubbins of my fingers. I had intended to have the photographer take a shot of our hands, and I certainly didn't want my disgusting nails to show. My friend and I lost patience finally, and I threw the nails back into the box. I lit another cigarette and, with it hanging from my mouth, I took our cups to the counter to refill them.

"Damn!" I cried out when I saw the strange car pull into our farmyard. Some of my fiancé's relatives had arrived. I grabbed my cigarette and drowned it under the faucet. This turned out to be my second attempt to quit smoking. It would last three days. By the time our honeymoon was partway over, I was sneaking cigarettes.

I don't recommend a honeymoon as a time to quit smoking, especially unbeknownst to one's spouse. Our honeymoon was less than the wondrous experience we had expected. I was in a constant state of withdrawal, and he was left to ponder my mood swings. Years later, when I finally told him, he said he had thought my frequent trips to restaurant restrooms were a bit strange, but he attributed them to nerves. I asked him if he hadn't suspected I was smoking. "No," he said, "it never occurred to me. I guess I'd heard that some brides tend to be weepy and emotional, but I do remember thinking at the time that this is a little extreme."

* * *

You Can't Relapse If You Never Really Quit

Relapse is difficult to define because there is no total agreement, first of all, as to what constitutes recovery from nicotine addiction. Some experts explain recovery as having begun with the establishment of a predetermined period of abstinence—whether it's two weeks, six months, or a year. If an addict resumes tobacco use after having lived without it for that specified time, it's a relapse. Others believe recovery isn't signified so much by a period of time, as by a state of mind. Is the addict's day-to-day existence relatively free of craving and obsession with tobacco, with no tobacco used? If so, that's recovery, and any resumption of use would be relapse. I favor the second of these definitions because, although I was abstinent for nearly eight months, I don't believe I'd ever begun genuine recovery. Cigarettes were still the center of my life; I just wasn't smoking them. I hadn't learned to cope with life without them.

People who have lived happily without cigarettes do relapse though. Circumstances may vary, but the explanation is the same for all addicts: relapse is always possible because the addiction is never gone. An alcoholic can be recovering, but not recovered. The addiction is always there, and the old alcoholic behavior is only one drink away. Recovery, for addicts, is discovering how to live without their drug of choice. For many, the danger of relapse seems unlikely as their lives become better and better. They may even begin to question whether they were true addicts, and with this questioning may come the wistful thought that it would be nice to be able to have a drink (or a cigarette or a snort) once in a while.

Although the wish to be like everybody else, to be "normal," is understandable, it's not possible. The choice isn't between abstinence and moderation; it's between recovery and relapse into the illness as deeply or more deeply than before.

Recovery doesn't mean recovery of the ability to drink, smoke, or use socially. What the addict recovers is the ability to make choices, rather than having them made by the addiction.

Addictive use becomes an instinctive behavior for a hard-core smoker. Put into high-stress situations, our instincts to use kick in. Abstinence reintroduces us to the pain, vulnerability, and fear we have handled with our drug, and each onset of high stress or dark feelings can trigger our desire for the drug. Even recovering smokers report cravings as much as five and ten years after quitting. These cravings are not constant, as they often are at the beginning of abstinence, but they are reminders of how strong the addiction is.

One recovering smoker says that it seemed he had the cravings whenever he did something he hadn't done as a non-smoker. During the hunting season after he had quit, he said he was nearly overcome by the craving and even thought about going to town to buy cigarettes. "It's almost as though I had to do everything over again as a nonsmoker to pattern myself into that mold," he says.

Sometimes relapse appears to be a more deliberate act in reaction to something or someone in the smoker's life. A woman, who was hurt by her husband, "chose" to start smoking again because she knew he hated it. The pain of losing someone triggers the memory of the numbing effect of nicotine in a smoker who justifies relapse to medicate what seems to be unbearable pain.

Most often, though, relapse arises from the belief (or wish) that smoking "just this once" won't hurt. Many of us smokers have found ourselves saying something like, "I can't believe how dumb I was. I had it beaten. Hadn't smoked for three years. Then one night I got together with some old friends and decided to smoke with them. I was hooked again just like that."

In his title essay from the book *Controversy and Other Essays in Journalism*, William Manchester describes his experiences when gathering material for *The Death of a President,* his book about the assassination of John F. Kennedy. Early on, he talks about his experience interviewing members of Kennedy's family:

> The research was difficult—about half the people I interviewed displayed deep emotional distress while trying to answer my questions—though none of the sessions were as affecting as those with Jackie. Future historians may be puzzled by odd clunking noises on the tapes. They were ice cubes. The only way we could get through those long evenings was with the aid of great containers of daiquiris. (Bobby wouldn't drink while being interviewed. His replies were abrupt, often monosyllabic—and much less responsive.) There are also frequent sound of matches being struck. Before our first taping I had carefully put the Wollensak recorder where I would see it and she wouldn't. I didn't want her to worry about the machine. Also, I had to be sure that the little light on it was winking, that the reels were turning, that all this wasn't being lost. It was a good plan. Its defect was revealed to me when she took the wrong chair. Then the only way I could check the light was by hunching up. It was an odd movement; I needed an excuse for it. A cigarette box on a low table provided one. Before the evening I hadn't smoked for two years. At the end of it I was puffing away, and eight more years would pass before I could quit again.

At times it may be our family or friends who help us relapse. They may be unprepared for a lengthy recovery process which may include uncontrolled outbursts of anger, depression, and a laundry list of physical and emotional symptoms. It's not that they don't love us. Their willingness (and sometimes encouragement) to have us return to smoking may be based on two factors. First, because they don't accept the concept of this being an addiction in the fullest sense of the word, they're unprepared for extreme withdrawal. Second, our abstinence, at least in the short run, is often more devastating to the family structure than our using was. With other addictions, the family is often more willing to endure the erratic behavior and mood swings of the recovering addict because the survival of the family is at stake and because no matter how difficult early recovery is, it is usually better and less stressful than when the drinking or the using was happening.

*   *   *

"When You Really Want to ..."

She listened to and encouraged me dozens of times in the months I struggled not to smoke. She had quit years earlier, and it had been hard for her, too, she told me. "Hang in there," she'd say. "It'll get better." She told me the things that had worked for her. "Keep busy." "Just don't smoke today."

I dreaded calling her and telling her I'd started smoking again. I felt like a child about to confess a wrongdoing, a failure. She had invested so much time in helping me. She'd listened to my sieges of anger and to the words of my deepening depression. Yet she would understand. Except for my immediate family, she knew better than anyone else how much I'd suffered. She knew how hard I'd tried.

Her voice was soft and loving, as it always was when we talked. And then I told her. "I started smoking again."

The soft, loving tone never wavered. There was none of the anger or recrimination I'd half feared. She was sorry, she told me, and then she said something that cut more than anger could have: "It's okay. You'll do it another time. You'll be able to quit when you really want to."

I learned two things from that phone call. One thing was about her—about a lot of nonsmokers really. The other was about myself. Neither was flattering. Her judgment of my attempt to quit was harsh and totally dependent on the outcome. If I successfully quit, that meant I *wanted* to. Lack of success meant I didn't want to. Whatever my withdrawal had been was of no significance to her. Her sympathy and encouragement had been sincere, I'm sure, but she had seen the withdrawal symptoms as being only something to endure. To her, the only determining factors of success were willpower and desire. Her statement told me flatly I hadn't enough of either.

Even more demoralizing was the discovery I made about

myself. In time, I came to understand that her message to me had been the same message I'd given others over the years. I had no sympathy for overweight people who didn't have enough pride to shape up. A little exercise and wise eating didn't seem too much to ask of them. I, a woman nearly five-foot-ten and 130 pounds, a woman who had always been thin, had shaken her head in dismay at others' seeming lack of willpower. Only after my sudden weight gain and my inability to control it, only after giving up my drug of choice and searching for nicotine's relief in food and alcohol — only then did I understand and have compassion for these other people.

I also understood my father better. Years earlier, submitting to pressure from his family, he had quit drinking for six months. Later he told me that he returned to drinking because he felt as though he was having a heart attack. I'd laughed to my husband and spit out my contempt: "The old fool! Who does he think he's kidding? A heart attack! He just was looking for an excuse to start drinking again." I didn't say he'd be able to quit when he really wanted to, but that's what I believed. I was still convinced his drinking was a choice. That he was angry by choice. That he had hurt me by choice.

Confronted with proof of my own addiction and the pain of withdrawal, I finally began to understand my father and his addiction. The "bad times" no longer dominated my growing up memories. I remembered the good times, too, and I felt loved. The weeping that had plagued me for the eight months of my withdrawal returned, but with a difference. Now it was brief; it was cleansing. I wept for the man who until then had died unmourned.

* * *

WHAT IT COMES DOWN TO

Coming Home

His wife and his two youngest children were with my father that morning when he died. Miles away, my family and I were taking down our Christmas decorations. I was just walking back into the house after having carried the tree outside when the phone began to ring. I snarled at my children as they instinctively headed for the phone. I'd answer it, I snapped, knowing at once the meaning of the call and not wanting my brother or sister to have to talk to a child at a time like this.

His voice was thin and hollow. "It's over," he said simply. There was little to say other than I would call my other brother and I was sure we'd be coming down later in the day.

We had been receiving daily reports, so my brother was prepared for my call. He agreed we should leave that day for our hometown. It was decided my children and I would come to his house and pick him up. I'd be leaving shortly, I told him, so we'd be "home" by suppertime. Within an hour, the children and I were ready to set off. Two hours later, my brother, my three children, and I left my brother's home and started off on what would become the most frightening experience of our lives.

To begin with, there was an eeriness about the trip itself. I drove along the route so familiar to all of us, yet everything seemed foreign. Partly, I suppose, it was due to the unusual silence within the car. My children rode quietly in the backseat with a few hushed comments here and there, but none of the bickering so common to them in the confines of the car—no familiar outcries of who could sit by the window or of who was crowding or of wanting to stop for food. They probably were keying off my brother and me. We, too, were subdued and broke the silence only occasionally with remote memories of our father or of our growing up years together.

The strangeness of the drive was further accentuated by the emptiness of the landscape as we approached the plains section of southern Minnesota. The bleakness of the January sky was an extension of the frozen farmland stretching out before us. The fields, covered by the most recent snowfall, had already become gray from the soil-laden winds. That day the winds were stronger than usual. Strips of snow, like drifting fog, snaked across the road before us. We heard and felt the wind as it hurled itself howling against the car. Only a few other travelers were on the road—unusual for this highway on a weekend.

I turned on the radio, partly to infuse the car with life and partly to hear the weather forecast. There was not a long wait; the weather obviously was making news. The cold weather—cold even by Minnesota standards—had been intensified by winds up to fifty miles per hour, and the radio announcer was reading a list of activities cancelled due to the arctic conditions. Following were the warnings we hear during every winter cold snap: stay indoors; if you must go out, dress warmly and cover exposed skin; carry emergency equipment if you travel by car; and on and on. The meteorologist was forecasting even colder temperatures by nightfall and "blowing and drifting snow." I signalled my left-hand turn from the four-lane highway and turned south onto a narrow state road. Our hometown was less than an hour and a half ahead.

The road's decline—made necessary to tie in the lower level state highway to the higher four-lane—is usually unnoticeable; the angle is so slight. That day we experienced it, foot by foot, as the visibility gradually worsened with our descent to the level of the farmland around. Within a mile, I had slowed to ten or fifteen miles per hour, and my brother and I were desperately scanning ahead to find either the center line or the white markings along the right side of the road. We had hit a ground blizzard—the snow blinding us was not falling snow, but the remnants of the last snowfall being whirled from the ground by the wind, creating a horizontal storm. Every so often, neither my brother nor I could find a guiding line, and we'd both be calling out, "I can't see it. I can't see it." Then I'd apply the brakes, stop, and wait until we could see a road marking. Several times when this happened, my brother asked, "Is the car moving?" The swirling snow had so disoriented us, we couldn't tell when we were moving and when we weren't. "Yes," I would assure him, and then to make doubly sure, I pushed harder on the brake, twice causing us to lurch forward in our seats.

We tried to estimate how far we'd driven in the storm and how much longer it would be before we reached the next town. I had a sudden sense of hopelessness. I just knew we were going to drift off the edge of the road blindly and that it would be hours or days before we were found frozen to death in the eighty-five below windchill.

My brother's thoughts were in tune with mine. "If we go into the ditch, we'll still be okay," he said. "This arctic gear I'm wearing is great. I'd be able to walk for help."

I said nothing in reply; we both knew this wasn't true. Our only chance would be to stay inside the car, huddling together and praying that help would come in time. Often, people who have deserted their cars to find help have died in storms like this. Disoriented, they may unknowingly walk in circles. Sometimes the tragedy seems even greater when we're told that the victim's body was found just a few feet from a farmhouse or within arm's length of the car that had been abandoned hours earlier. *No,* I thought, *if the worst happens, we'll stay together.*

The children leaned forward, their bodies and voices tense as they tried to help us spot the marks along the road. Did they know how serious this was, or were they reacting to my fear? I was upset with myself for having brought them, risking their lives like that. I raged against myself for packing the survival kit in the trunk, instead of the backseat where it belonged. My thoughts raced in terror: *If we went into the ditch, could I safely retrieve the blankets and gear from the trunk? Would I dare risk turning the ignition off to take the keys? Would I lose my way in those few short steps to the back of the car? What if I dropped the keys?* Then a new fear hit me: *How many cigarettes did I have left in this pack? How many did my brother have?*

I never had to discover whether I would have chanced a trip to the trunk to retrieve cigarettes and other necessities. An hour and a half and a mere fifteen miles later, we crept into a small town. The buildings and trees acted as windbreaks, and visibility was fine within the town. We drove to a private home with inviting lights. The kind people there fed us and called the pastor of a nearby church, and we slept that night in sleeping bags on the church basement floor.

It may be that my senses were heightened by the impact of my father's death. Or perhaps the terror of knowing how easily and quickly my loved ones and I could have perished served to sharpen my awareness. I'm not sure, but in hindsight I think my view of smoking began to change that day. It suddenly didn't make any sense. I had seriously considered risking my life for a pack of cigarettes. Why was it so important?

That evening, passing a few hours in the church before it was time to sleep, I should have been overwhelmed with a sense of peace and thanksgiving. Instead, I was jumpy and anxious from lack of nicotine. The pastor's only request in opening his church to us was that we not smoke there. We had agreed. The large building was taking a long time to warm up in the severe cold. But we were safe, and the children were sleeping. Outside, the temperatures continued to plunge and the winds were still heavy. No one could survive long outdoors on a night like that.

My brother and I often talk about the close call we had on the day our father died. We remark on the kindness of the people and laugh at our promise not to smoke in the church.

I tell him it was then that I realized I had lost control of my life. Though I maintained pretense of control by keeping my promise not to smoke inside, I willingly stood outdoors, shivering and smoking with my brother as the brutal north wind whistled through the crackling trees.

* * *

Not Normal

Despite how much like everyone else we nicotine addicts may act and sound, our behavior is not normal. When a person's decisions are almost constantly influenced by the need for a drug, it only stands to reason he or she will do some strange things. No matter how hungry we all had been the night we were stranded in the blizzard, it would not have made sense to any of us to walk anywhere to get food. Had someone asked me to, I—like any normal person—would have refused to risk exposure to those temperatures. Where my smoking behavior is concerned, however, normal reactions do not apply.

Little of what I do makes sense except as the behavior of an addict. Yet, because tobacco use is, for the most part, accepted as normal, my peculiar behavior as a smoker is rarely questioned. Had I walked through a blizzard to a bar, most people would have had no trouble labeling my behavior as unusual—certainly not that of a normal drinker. Because it was nicotine I needed, my smoking outdoors in sub-zero weather is likely to be viewed as amusing or, at worst, eccentric.

It may be that before intervention can happen with the same effectiveness for us smokers as it does for alcoholics and other drug addicts, more nonsmokers need to recognize that we have a disease. No matter what we nicotine addicts claim to the contrary, much of our behavior is controlled or, at the very least, influenced by our need to maintain a certain level of nicotine in our systems.

The word *need* implies something that is essential to life. We all need food. We all need love. We all need protection from the elements. We don't need chocolate cake or Hawaiian vacations. Yet as a smoker I *need* a cigarette. I make and act upon this statement as an irrefutable truth. I smoke in inappropriate places and at inappropriate times. I smoke when I know other people wish I wouldn't. I smoke when I know it's hurting others. Frequently, if others complain of burning eyes or of smoke irritating a cold, I feel angry or martyred. I think of them as being the inconsiderate ones. After all, they know I need a cigarette.

Most needs can almost always be delayed if necessary. Even when people are very hungry, they will postpone eating until the guests arrive or until the children get home from after-school activities. I rarely postpone smoking, and when I do it's usually with extreme agitation or emotional upset. What I really need is to satisfy my craving, the insatiable voice of my addiction.

The one overriding value for an addicted smoker is: cigarettes come first. When I ignore other people's needs and comfort, I don't believe it's because I don't love them. It's that my addiction very often demands immediate satisfaction to the exclusion of everyone and everything else.

This may be revealed in a range of behaviors from simple delaying actions ("I'll be with you in a minute" or "I'll read to you when I'm done") to a complete abdication of responsibility because of my inability to subject myself to an extended period of abstinence. I have declined chaperoning my children at church or school activities because of the time required without access to my cigarettes. An hour—two, at the most—is my limit, and whatever the activity, I'm not available.

On one level, nothing is of more value for me than participating in my children's lives. But at the level of my addiction, where these day-to-day decisions are played out, what I claim to be my real values will be drowned out by *cigarettes come first*. When my children were small, one would occasionally creep up and cuddle next to me. Invariably, another would toddle in and demand to sit with me too. I can clearly remember telling the child, "Come on and climb up here next to your brother (sister). There's no room next to Mommy." So why didn't I just move the first child and myself over to make room on the other side of me? The answer's easy, and painful to admit: I *always* sit next to an end table to accommodate my smoking paraphernalia.

*   *   *

Distancing

Some emotional distancing is required to avoid the pain of facing the impact of our unloving actions on others. This brings our addiction full circle as we use nicotine to dull our sense of failure, guilt, fear, and anger.

In discussions with other smokers, I've mentioned the sadness I often experience in late evenings. The feeling accompanies the "last" cigarette of the day. As it gradually burns down, I feel a combination of panic and loneliness. I often decide, *Well, I'll just have another cigarette after this one*, and the negative feelings disappear. This practice—especially when it's repeated several times in an evening—often makes me the last one up at night. I can always find a "logical" reason for staying up: a project to finish, a movie to watch, or "I just want to finish reading this chapter." On the surface, these are all true, but the deeper motive is permission to smoke longer and later. I've been amazed at how many other smokers have said they do the same thing. This confirms many smokers' description of themselves as loners, and further demonstrates emotional distancing through physical distancing, not to mention the intimacy issues implied.

The smoke itself can be a tangible wall—a smoke screen—physically distancing us from nonsmokers. Even after the smoke has cleared, the lingering smell on my breath and clothing acts as an invisible wall between me and others. I, and many smokers like me, can know these things and yet continue with our irrational behavior as if it is the rest of the world that is out of step.

How hungry would I have to be before I would eat from a garbage can? I like to think I would have to be starving, desperate. Yet I have dug through car ashtrays and garbage bags when I've run out of cigarettes. I've been thrilled with the discovery of half-smoked butts covered with coffee grounds and who knows what else. I've dried them out with lighters and hair dryers, then happily smoked them. I've made dozen of trips outside and sat in the cold car waiting for the lighter to heat up, after running out of matches. I once hit upon the idea of using my husband's acetylene torch. I dug through cupboards, shelves, and tool boxes before I found it, only to discover it required a match to light it.

I'm not alone in these bizarre behaviors. Many of us have

- gone out at midnight to buy cigarettes to assure a morning's supply.
- stayed up after everyone has gone to bed, smoked the only three cigarettes left in our house or apartment, and then gone out at midnight to buy a pack.
- "borrowed" cigarettes from complete strangers. (I can't imagine leaning over to another patron in a restaurant and saying, "Excuse me, but could I have a few of your French fries? I'm all out.")
- ignored evidence of children's smoking because we don't want to be reminded of our own.
- quickly put out a cigarette before someone enters the room so we could light a fresh one right away and thereby conceal our heavy smoking.

* * *

No Bargain

Most smokers with many years behind them have at least the beginnings of cigarette-related health conditions. It could be a cough; almost all of us have one. There's probably short-windedness or a heavy feeling after climbing steps or with other exertions. Many of us have gradually become less active over the years of our addiction. This may be due to a natural avoidance of activities that preclude smoking—water sports, running, tennis, skiing, or others requiring intense or two-handed participation. Part of our lessening of activity could be a natural result of lower energy levels.

For many of us, the haunting fear of cancer or heart disease is a nearly constant presence, especially as we move into our forties and fifties—ages at which people we've known have died. The illusion of our youth—that we had almost endless years ahead and that the loss of a few years was not such a big deal—suddenly *is* a big deal because a few years represents a substantial part of our future.

When we face these fears, we often bargain with a faceless, whimsical fate. When I began smoking, I thought people who were in their late forties—my present age—were old and the best part of their lives were gone. Today, I try to strike a bargain: if I could live to my father's age—seventy—I would be happy. But then I remember my father's words: "I wish I could have two more years with you." Perhaps we're always bargaining for more, hoping to escape the very real dangers our addiction exposes us to. For many smokers, the acknowledgment of those dangers is enough to break through their denial and lead them to the help they need. But for me, and many other addicted smokers, the bargaining continues.

I believe most smokers are at least vaguely aware of not being free, of being tied to illogical and self-defeating behaviors. There's often a sense of "I'm better than this" and even more often "I wish I were better than this." The hard truth of addiction flashes before us from time to time and feeds the old fears of being different from, weaker than, or morally inferior to others. A sense of self-sufficiency and of being in harmony with the rest of the world may elude us then. Dictated to by a drug, we've avoided risks because we've feared failure; we've not reached out because we've been too tightly curled up within ourselves. And we've not developed living skills because our drug was taking care of us. In a word, we've not *grown*.

A kind of spiritual bankruptcy is a natural result of addiction, as a drug becomes the overwhelming power in our lives. It becomes a god of sorts. It never fails. It is always there. And it protects us from whatever we haven't wanted to deal with. This, for me and many others, is difficult to give up. Perhaps the commitment to recovery comes with the realization that what we've been living is not real. The world is not always safe, fair, or predictable. People are not always kind. To depend on the protection of a drug, however, doesn't change the world or the people in it. It only alters our perception of it, which means we're forever playing "let's pretend" like children.

* * *

Creating Solitude

The friendship is one of those that seemed to spring up quickly in full bloom with none of the tentative steps most relationships seem to follow. A love of books, I suppose, and words was the bond. Talking as we did so often about them led naturally to self-revelation. The friendship was just suddenly there, and neither of us questioned it.

Our conversation that night had focused on the need for solitude. He had been feeling pressed in by demands of school and career and had an aching need for time alone, and there was none. He'd asked if I understood what he was feeling. And yes, I did, I told him, but because of the busy household I live in, I've had to find solitude within a hurricane. I told him about the speaker at a writers' conference who had been emphatic about the writer's need for solitude. That writer, who is married to another writer, had found it by building a home in a remote, rustic setting. There, they had established a writing routine—specific hours set aside for creating in silence.

"That sounds so ideal," I told my friend, "but for most of us it isn't realistic. Some of us chose to have children, and no children I know are impressed by their parents' need for solitude, much less silence. So I often write amidst uproar, accepting the questions, arguments, phone calls, and other people's schedules."

"But then you never find solitude."

"You know, I think I do. I just realized that with all this going on around me, I'm often able to feel solitude—even isolation. I never thought about it like this before, but I think I use the nicotine to shut myself off from the uproar, no matter how noisy or disrupting it might seem to anyone else. I'll have to remember to use that in the book."

We talked then for a while about my writing, about this

book. And after a few minutes, I apologized for again directing the conversation to the subject. "I'm really sorry, but it seems like that's all I think about. And it's not just the book. I've been so wrapped up in this for so long—for years it was the smoking, now it's the book, and, above all, it's the wanting to quit smoking."

"Do you think you can ever let go of it?" His voice was filled with concern. "What I mean is, I really hope you can quit—for yourself, for me, and your other friends. But if you can't, do you think you can get on with your life? What it comes down to is, can you just say, 'I've tried and it hasn't worked. I accept myself as a smoker'?"

This was something I'd never thought about before, but in an instant I thought he was right. "Yes, I can. I'll have to." The thought seemed freeing. I'd no longer have to be looking, and searching, and hoping. *When the writing's done, I'll try one last time,* I told myself. *And then it will be over, no matter what the outcome is.*

* * *

Coming to a Decision

"Did you know," I asked my daughter one evening, "that women seem to have more difficulty quitting smoking or any other addiction?"

Her angry response caught me by surprise. "I think all you're trying to do is make excuses for your smoking," she told me. "All this does is give you reasons for not quitting. You keep talking about it being an addiction, and then you don't have to quit. It bothers me, Mom. It really does, and I think you could quit if you'd just stick to it longer. I know you feel unhappy when you quit, but it wouldn't last forever, you know."

"How do I know that?"

"Because. You know it would have to end sometime. Even if it took a year – or two years – so what would it matter? Why can't you just say, 'Even if it takes two years, I'm going to make it'?"

"Because," I told her, "I *don't* know that it would end, even in two years – or four – or ten. I don't know if the withdrawal and the depression would ever end."

It's only natural our two perceptions of my smoking would be different. She can't understand the power addiction has over my life. What she sees is, me smoking. What she believes is, every time I light a cigarette, I'm choosing to smoke, to offend her, to risk the health of my family, to tempt the statistics that say I am needlessly shortening my life and courting an agonizing death. Her feelings are hurt by what she understands to be my callousness toward her wishes and our health. More recently, she stated her feelings very clearly: "I'm not worried about myself, Mom. I just don't want you to die. I don't want to lose you."

How can I expect her to understand? I've smoked for nearly thirty years, but only for the last seven have I actually thought of smoking as an addiction. Only for this relatively short time have I seen how perfectly smoking mirrors the behavior of alcoholics and other addicts. Only now do I recognize the sad similarity between her pleas and my asking my father to quit drinking. And only recently have I come to understand why my father appears so frequently in what I've written about my smoking.

Throughout these months, I've been troubled by the frequent references to him and his alcoholism. My daughter has challenged me on this: "Why do you keep talking about Grandpa and his drinking? You're supposed to be writing about smoking." I've worried that she's right. Have I been making excuses for my addiction by laying the blame at his feet? Have I set myself up as a victim, a dramatic heroine, of a sad tale about a poor little girl whose father's alcoholism caused her to drift into another addiction? I've wondered and worried about this. But no more.

My father belongs here for many reasons, but primarily it's the irony that his drinking, the object of my obsession for so many years, was not the cause of his death. Above all, there's a sad wryness in understanding that the very cause of the anger and alienation between my father and me is also an undeniable bond. Perhaps stronger even than blood and our close physical resemblance is the bond of addiction. My story could just as well be my father's; both are about chemical dependency. And because I understand that now, I understand my father better.

From childhood into adulthood, I defined my father by his addiction. Or, more accurately, I defined him in terms of the symptoms of his addiction. I believed him to be an angry, unpredictable, frightening man. I believed he had caused the shame, embarrassment, and fear in my life. The symptoms of alcoholism created a chasm between us. Now, years later, I find myself by his side and realize we shared the same demons and even faced them in many of the same ways. His fears and vulnerability were diminished by alcohol and nicotine. I imagined mine safely held at bay with nicotine, and when deprived of it—especially during my longest abstinence of eight months—I used alcohol and food to fill the panicky emptiness. As I tried to eat and drink my way to a happy, nonsmoking state, it never occurred to me that my behavior was that of a chemically dependent person. In my mind, I was just doing what I could to cope. And coping, of course, is exactly what my father had done.

Living without nicotine is still my goal, but I no longer believe I'll reach it by simply not smoking. I've tried in recent months to stop smoking without using other drugs or compulsive behaviors such as overeating. Each time, I found myself looking for instant recovery, hoping to be cured. Recovery to me has meant everything would stay the same, except that I'm not smoking. But now I'm realizing that something more than abstinence is needed. I'm beginning to see that my addiction is not just a part of my life; it pervades it. I've been trying to free myself of the drug without making any other changes. Abstinence leaves me without nicotine, but still living with the old beliefs and behaviors that cry for the drug—in short, living a "dry drunk." Like any other addict, what I need is to make the changes necessary for living drug-free.

And I don't have to do it alone. Nicotine addiction is being taken more seriously today than in the past. Research supports what many of us smokers have been saying for years: "There's more to this than just quitting." Long-term support groups are being formed by members of cessation programs after the sessions end. Smokers Anonymous groups are growing and becoming more active. Some chemical dependency counselors are treating nicotine addiction with the same methods used for other drug abuse problems. A few inpatient treatment programs of one to two weeks are now available for smokers, and it seems likely that their number will grow as more people accept the reality of hard-core nicotine addiction.

I don't have choice and power over my addiction. But I do have the power to hate the smoking, and I can choose to act on that hatred by asking for help. I understand that there are no guarantees or easy answers. I will never be free of my addiction—I can never be a nonaddict—but I owe it to myself, my family, and my father to grasp any chance I have for recovery. I was mistaken to tell my friend that yes, I could go on with my life and accept myself as a smoker. I no longer can.

* * *

Appendix*

Quitting Tips

- With the aid of a physician, investigate the possibility of using a nicotine gum to help you abstain from tobacco. The gum is intended to be a temporary aid in coping with the early stages of nicotine withdrawal. Be aware, though, that it may become a replacement addiction.
- Look for a good smoking cessation program to enroll in.
- Find out if there is a Smokers Anonymous group in your area and begin attending a few meetings.
- Tap into everything you've learned about recovery from addiction in other Twelve Step programs.
- Start working each Step of the program and develop a strong relationship with your Higher Power.
- Find a sponsor, someone who has quit using tobacco and can offer you support when you need it.
- Avoid perfectionism in breaking the habit.
- Identify your tobacco use patterns; choose one pattern a week, and break it (put off that first cigarette in the morning; quit smoking in meetings, in the car, after meals, on the phone).
- Don't quit forever—just quit for one day at a time.
- Tell your family, friends, and co-workers that you are quitting.
- Make smoking each cigarette a decision—bring it to your conscious mind, rather than let it be the unthinking, repetitive behavior it has become.
- Pick a day to quit—and quit. It's time to enjoy life!

---

*Reprinted from the Hazelden pamphlet, *Twelve Steps for Tobacco Users: For Recovering People Addicted to Nicotine,* by Jeanne E.

Additional Help

Though some people can learn to abstain from nicotine use by themselves, many of us need help to quit and to maintain abstinence. The surgeon general's 1988 report has outlined some useful information about what kinds of treatment can help, in what ways, and why. The following summary will allow you to assess the kind of help you might need, and to evaluate the various smoking cessation programs available in your area.

Two Goals of Treatment

First, keep in mind that there are two primary goals of treatment for nicotine addiction:

- *To stop smoking,* or to eliminate use of the substance you are dependent upon, whether it is cigarettes or other forms of tobacco
- *To avoid relapse,* or to maintain your abstinence from the use of nicotine

The important thing to remember regarding the first goal—to stop using nicotine—is that setting a goal of merely reducing your intake is not helpful; no level of cigarette smoking or ingestion of other tobacco products is safe.

The second goal—avoiding relapse—is vital to recovery because factors that contribute to nicotine use operate for many years after nicotine use ceases. Ongoing factors such as stress and exposure to people and places associated with nicotine use create continual invitations to relapse.

The best treatment approaches contain both physiological (smoking cessation) and behavioral (maintenance of abstinence) components. These help you achieve an immediate goal of stopping tobacco use while giving you new skills to cope with ongoing behavioral and environmental pressures.

Treatment Approaches

To recover from nicotine addiction, the first thing you must do is stop using the drug. To help you do this, you might consider using a replacement drug like nicotine gum. The use of nicotine gum reduces the need for your primary nicotine source and reduces drug-seeking, or nicotine-seeking, behavior. Though the urge to smoke or use other forms of tobacco will not disappear, withdrawal symptoms will be reduced or eliminated, allowing you to maintain normal social and work responsibilities while you quit using tobacco. Thus, the use of a replacement or substitute such as nicotine gum can help you address some of the physiological problems associated with nicotine addiction. Nicotine gum requires a prescription, so consult with your physician before using it.

Treatment approaches that will help you make necessary behavior changes take many forms. Programs might combine individual, group, and family counseling with skills training and buddy support systems.

Because maintaining abstinence is such a major goal, it is important to find a treatment program that offers skills training in several areas. According to the surgeon general's report, people who have developed skills in the areas of relapse prevention, leisure activities, stress management, and social support are best able to maintain abstinence from nicotine.

- *Relapse prevention skills* include training in assertiveness, social skills, and problem-solving, and practice in handling high-risk situations.
- *Leisure skills* involve learning or relearning relaxation activities, particularly physical activities and exercise.
- *Stress management skills* involve learning to deal with negative emotions associated with difficult events or relationships.

- *Social support skills* help you find support from friends, family, support groups, counselors, peers, or sponsors to help you maintain ongoing abstinence.

Where to Go for Help

Now that you know what to look for in treatment approaches, you will want to contact a specific program. Your doctor may suggest a program he or she is familiar with. You can also look in The Yellow Pages under "Smoking Cessation" or "Smokers" for a list of treatment programs available in your area. Many hospitals also have programs; if you are familiar with a particular hospital, call and ask if they offer a smoking cessation program. Recognized organizations—the American Lung Association, the American Cancer Society, and the American Heart Foundation—offer smoking cessation programs. Contact the state headquarters of any of these organizations for program information.

And, to find out if there is a Smokers Anonymous group in your area, call the national hot line at (415) 922-8575.

References and Notes

Page

11 Steven J. Levy, *Managing the Drugs in Your Life: A Commonsense Personal and Family Guide* (New York: McGraw-Hill Book Co., 1983), 123–24.

12 *The Health Consequences of Smoking: Nicotine Addiction* (Rockville, Md.: U.S. Department of Health and Human Services, 1988), 9.

22-25 *Introducing . . . Smokers Anonymous* (San Francisco: Smokers Anonymous World Services, 1988).

31 *The Health Consequences of Smoking*, 255–56.

44 Dolly D. Gahagan, *Switch Down and Quit* (Berkeley, Calif.: Ten Speed Press, 1987), 115.

61-62 Craig Nakken, *The Addictive Personality* (Center City, Minn.: Hazelden Educational Materials, 1988), 5.

64 M. Scott Peck, *The Road Less Traveled* (New York: Simon & Schuster, Inc., 1978), 16.

66 Peck, *The Road Less Traveled*, 16.

69 Nakken, *The Addictive Personality*, 17.

90-91 William Manchester, *Controversy and Other Essays in Journalism 1950–1975* (Boston: Little, Brown and Company, 1976), 11–12. Reprinted with permission.